HUMAN DEVELOPMENT NETWORK
Health, Nutrition, and Population Series

Health, Nutrition, and Population Indicators

A Statistical Handbook

Eduard Bos
Vivian Hon
Akiko Maeda
Gnanaraj Chellaraj
Alexander Preker

The World Bank
Washington, D.C.

© 1999 The International Bank for Reconstruction
and Development / THE WORLD BANK
1818 H Street, N.W.
Washington, D.C. 20433, U.S.A.

All rights reserved
Manufactured in the United States of America
First printing December 1998

Cover graphic by Supon Design Group, Washington, D.C.

Library of Congress Cataloging-in-Publication Data

Health, nutrition, and population indicators : a statistical handbook
  / Eduard Bos … [et al.].
        p.   cm. — (Health, nutrition, and population series)
     Includes bibliographical references.
     ISBN 0-8213-4184-7
     1. Health status indicators—Statistics—Handbooks, manuals, etc.
2. Medical statistics—Handbooks, manuals, etc.   3. Health—
Statistics—Handbooks, manuals, etc.   4. Nutrition—Statistics—
Handbooks, manuals, etc.   5. Population—Statistics—Handbooks,
manuals, etc.   I. Bos, Eduard R.   II. Series.
RA407.H437   1998
614.4'2'021—dc21   98-30586
                                                                    CIP

Contents

Abstract

This statistical handbook is an up-to-date compilation of indicators of levels and trends in health status, health determinants, health systems, and health finance. The first sections highlight trends in health indicators and then analyze and explain the trends. The last section contains statistical tables, with data presented by country, region, and income group. A summary of data sources and a list of definitions follows the tables.

During the past few decades trends in health status have shown vast improvements in life expectancy, malnutrition, and fertility decline. However, improvements in health have been unequally distributed, both geographically and among income groups. The trends also show a shift in the burden of disease from infectious to noncommunicable diseases and injuries. New diseases, such as AIDS, and re-emerging ones, such as tuberculosis, will figure prominently among the remaining infectious diseases.

Trends in health systems and health finance indicate that the financing and delivery of HNP services in many low-income countries is carried out by the private sector. Large discrepancies exist among countries in the amounts spent on health, with per capita expenditures almost 1,000-fold greater in some high-income countries than in low-income countries. Recently, a number of middle-income countries have started to face the challenge of rapidly rising health expenditures in both the public and private sectors, which lead to fiscally unsustainable health systems.

The indicators in the tables:
- Identify countries that have and have not made progress in reducing mortality and morbidity for vulnerable groups
- Reveal the importance of different conditions and diseases in different countries
- Identify low-income countries that are not spending enough to finance a minimum level of essential health services, as well as middle-income countries that have high and unsustainable public health expenditures
- Identify factors associated with poor HNP outcomes.

The limitations of the data are pointed out in the text. Considerable uncertainty about the reliability and validity of basic health status and health finance data is often the result of insufficient government commitment to data collection. International agencies, such as the World Bank, should consider supporting capacity building in data collection.

Foreword

A major objective of work in the health, nutrition, and population (HNP) sector is to improve health outcomes. To monitor and evaluate progress toward this objective, the Bank needs to improve its own and borrower capacity to measure health outcomes as well as the performance of health systems and the state of health finance.

The overview and tables in this volume summarize health outcomes, systems, and finance nationally, regionally, and globally. By providing key indicators in the HNP sector, the tables document progress made over the past decades and provide a baseline from which to measure future changes.

This volume is intended to provide a comparative perspective on country performance and to point to future challenges in the health sector. For many countries, economic and health sector indicators are missing or of poor quality, which indicates the need both to develop more effective indicators and to include monitoring and evaluation components in project design.

This volume is part of the process of developing and implementing the Bank's health, nutrition, and population sector strategy. Efforts to monitor impacts and outcomes are a key priority of the strategy.

Christopher Lovelace
Acting Director
Health, Nutrition, and
  Population Department

David de Ferranti
Vice President
Human Development
  Network

Acknowledgments

The material in this volume was prepared as part of the World Bank's health, nutrition, and population sector strategy during 1996–97. It was undertaken by the HNP Family of the Human Development Network under the guidance of the HNP Sector Board.

Many individuals contributed to this study by bringing reports and data to our attention that we would have missed otherwise. Others reviewed the material or provided useful suggestions and comments on the selection of indicators. The authors would like to thank the following individuals in particular: Richard G. A. Feachem, Mariam Claeson, Timothy Heleniak, Dean Jamison, Nicole Klingen, Ellen Lukens, Sulekha Patel, Dena Ringold, Claudia Rokx, George Schieber, Laura Shrestha, Ruben Suarez, and Diana Weil.

Overview

The World Bank has compiled up-to-date and reliable indicators of levels and trends in health status, health determinants, health systems, and health finance as part of its work in the health, nutrition, and population (HNP) sector. A selection of these indicators was presented in the *Health, Nutrition, and Population Sector Strategy,* published by the World Bank in 1997.

This statistical handbook expands on the data presented in the *HNP Sector Strategy.* It presents a more complete set of indicators, as well as further analyses and explanations. It also highlights trends in important human development indicators used by the World Bank and the United Nations to monitor the impact of development programs.

The first section of this handbook is an overview of key HNP developments and trends. It begins with a summary of the major trends identified in the Bank's 1997 *HNP Sector Strategy,* as well as the major policy directions recommended as part of the strategy. This overview is followed by a general discussion of HNP data issues, including the role of indicators in implementing and monitoring the sector strategy, data sources and limitations, and the statistical methods used to construct some of the indicators. The first section concludes with a summary of the key findings revealed by the tables in this handbook.

The second section consists of the statistical tables, with data presented by country, region, and income group. A summary of data sources and definitions follows the tables.

This handbook is part of a series of World Bank HNP reports that are an outgrowth of the process of developing and implementing the Bank's sector strategy. The data are also available in electronic format. A future report in this HNP series will address Bank involvement in the HNP sector and operational indicators on performance of lending, economic and sector work, and research. For more information on this series, contact:

HNP Advisory Services, World Bank
1818 H Street, N.W., Washington, D.C., 20433
tel: (202) 473-2256; fax: (202) 522-3489.

Global Health Trends

Trends in Health Status

Advances in HNP during the past few decades have been impressive. During the second half of the twentieth century, life expectancy at birth for the world's population increased by almost 20 years, with an even greater increase among the populations of developing countries. The proportion of children who now die before reaching age five is less than half the level of 1960. Hundreds of millions of people in low- and middle-income countries are on the threshold of an era in which they will be safe from some of the world's most threatening diseases. Immunization now saves approximately 3 million children annually, and better control of diarrhea saves more than 1 million a year.

Economic progress during the past century has contributed significantly to health advances. Nutrition has improved through higher agricultural outputs and the introduction of a more varied diet, cutting child malnutrition rates in low- and middle-income countries by 20 percentage points.

The slowing of population growth rates has also had a positive impact. The global fertility rate (the average number of children born per woman) is now three, down from five at mid-century. Some low- and middle-income countries have reached replacement fertility levels of around two children per family as a result of better access to family planning as well as rising incomes and better education. More than half of all couples in low- and middle-income countries are now using contraception to plan their families.

While these overall gains in health status have been significant, many issues remain. Improvements in health have been unequally distributed, both geographically and among income groups. Of the total global disease burden, 93 percent is concentrated in low- and middle-income countries. The world's poorest populations continue to suffer from malnutrition, childhood infections, poor maternal and perinatal health, and high fertility. A total of 2 million deaths in children occur annually due to vaccine-preventable diseases; 200 million children under the age of five still suffer from malnutrition and anemia; and 30 percent of the world is still without safe water and sanitation. Furthermore, 120 million couples still lack options in family planning. Because of poor maternal health services, close to half a million women die each year from pregnancy-related causes.

Shifts in the disease burden from infectious to noncommunicable diseases and injuries—in part the result of changes in the age structure, and in part the result of changes in living conditions—require different approaches in prevention and care. New diseases such as AIDS, reemerging ones such as tuberculosis, and the development of drug-resistant microbes and parasites will figure prominently among the remaining infectious diseases.

Rapid population growth remains a major development challenge in many poor countries and places a heavy burden on health care and social services. Even as fertility gradually declines in many countries, the number of births will exceed the number of deaths for several more decades as a result of demographic momentum built into young population age structures. The world's population is projected to increase from 5.8 billion in 1997 to 9.2 billion in 2050, with over 95 percent of this increase occurring in low- and middle-income countries.

Trends in Health Systems

In most high-income countries—and many middle-income countries—governments have become central to social policy and health care, for both equity and efficiency reasons. In contrast, in many low-income countries, financing and delivery of HNP services remains largely in the private sector. In many of these countries, large segments of the poor still have no access to basic or effective care. In some other low-income countries, government-run health systems perform poorly, providing low-quality care resulting in poor outcomes.

The optimal balance between public and private involvement in the health sector varies from country to country, and is different in the case of financing from that in the case of service delivery. Many recent reforms have focused on correcting inequities and inefficiencies that occur when the balance between government and private sector roles becomes distorted in one direction or another. Governments in countries that have introduced successful reforms have often increased their role in providing health information, regulations, mandates, and financing, while fostering a more balanced participation of local communities, nongovernmental organizations, and the private sector in service delivery.

Trends in Health Finance

Global spending on health care was about US$2,330 billion in 1994 (9 percent of global GDP), making it one of the largest sectors in the world economy. While 84 percent of the world's population lives in low- and middle-income countries, these countries account for only 11 percent of global health spending. Poor countries tend to spend less on health not only on a per capita basis, but also as a percentage of GDP. This is reflected in the large differences in the proportion of national GDP spent on health—from under 1 percent in some countries to 15 percent in the United States. Per capita health expenditures (public and private) vary almost 1,000-fold among countries: from around US$3 to $5 per capita in some low-income countries such as Mali to $3,600 per capita in the United States.

Low personal income and low tax collection capacity in some countries help explain these wide discrepancies. Lack of financing usually translates into low levels of capital stocks such as beds, as well as of human resources such as doctors and nurses. Even

where capital stock is more adequate on a national basis, inequitable resource distribution may lower access to services by the poor.

Recently, a growing number of countries have started to face a different challenge: rapidly rising health expenditures in both the public and private sectors. Often public spending is forced above what is fiscally sustainable, and new spending goes to ineffective, inefficiently managed, low-quality care. The reasons for these increases include the escalating cost of medical technology, the increase in the burden of chronic diseases, rising popular expectations, and the growth of fee-for-service and third-party insurance. However, increased spending on health care alone does not necessarily improve HNP outcomes.

Health Policy Directions

Policymakers in low- and middle-income countries face difficult challenges caused by continued poverty, malnutrition, high fertility, and emerging and reemerging diseases; poor performance of many health systems; and inadequate or unsustainable health care financing, or both. Based on the trends summarized above, the World Bank's HNP sector strategy recommends that countries emphasize the following priorities to preserve past gains and address future threats in the health sector:

- *Improve HNP outcomes for the poor through targeted approaches.* This involves identifying poor individuals, households, and regions that are most vulnerable to illness, malnutrition, and high fertility.
- *Enhance the performance of HNP services.* The recommended strategy for public delivery of HNP services includes improving equity in access, raising efficiency in the use of scarce resources, improving the effectiveness of interventions, and raising the quality of care. The sector strategy also recommends a more balanced mix of public and private involvement in the HNP sector and calls for country-specific approaches to determine the optimal degree of government involvement.
- *Improve health care financing.* The HNP sector strategy recommends risk pooling as a fundamental aspect of social protection in the HNP sector. There

is also a need for governments to secure adequate levels of financing to provide essential public health activities and other essential HNP services. In low-income countries total government revenues may be insufficient to finance a minimum level of preventive and essential clinical services, and governments may need to mobilize additional financing from community sources and international donors. In middle-income countries governments can usually provide these services and may consider issues such as cost containment and equity and efficiency in the collection of revenues.

Data Issues

The Role of Indicators

Measurable indicators of health status, health systems, and health finance are indispensable to the analysis of problems in the HNP sector and to the improvement of health outcomes. Indicators can to provide information on inputs (that is, how much a country is spending on public health), on process or intermediate outcomes (that is, what proportion of the population has access to health services), and on impact (that is, how much health status has improved). These indicators also make it possible to implement and monitor the World Bank's HNP sector strategy as well as broader developmental goals in this sector.

The development and implementation of a broad HNP strategy (or other strategic plan) requires different indicators than those used in specific HNP projects to monitor project performance. Good indicators for monitoring implementation of a sector strategy are those that are relevant to the objectives of the strategy, those that are available for and comparable across a large number of low- and middle-income countries, those that are reliably measured through surveys or other empirical instruments, and those that can be linked with policies and projects.

In reality, few available HNP indicators fully satisfy these criteria. Improving HNP outcomes for the poor—one of the HNP strategy's main priorities—requires health status indicators for different income groups within countries. For most countries, however, these are unavailable and average income levels (GNP per capita) are used as a proxy. Similarly, the performance of health care systems is generally monitored through trends in access and outcomes rather than by direct indicators of efficacy and accountability.

In many countries impact indicators such as life expectancy estimates are not always based on accurate recording, but rather on extrapolations from or interpolations between surveys and censuses. Models, such as model life tables, are frequently used to derive information from incomplete data. Levels and trends in nutrition and access to health services are based on surveys that at times use very different definitions or that may be several years old. Monitoring trends in overall health expenditures is difficult because many countries lack regular household expenditure surveys that can measure private health expenditure.

Despite these limitations, the indicators used to evaluate the HNP sector will assist in implementing and monitoring the sector strategy by:

- Identifying which countries have and which have not made rapid progress in reducing mortality and morbidity for vulnerable groups, such as infants, children, and women.

- Revealing the importance of different conditions and diseases in order to answer such questions as: In which countries does malnutrition contribute to ill health? Where are high fertility and reproductive health issues most pressing? In which countries has adult mortality been increasing?

- Identifying low-income countries that are not spending enough to finance a minimum level of preventive and essential clinical services, and middle-income countries that are on a path to unsustainable expansion of public health expenditures.

- Identifying factors associated with poor HNP outcomes and issues that may become threats to future HNP outcomes and financing, for instance: In which countries are poverty and lack of social development a major threat? Where is public spending high while outcomes are poor? Which countries have rapidly aging populations? Where will emerging diseases such as HIV strike hardest, and in which countries are chronic diseases increasing most rapidly?

The indicators in the tables help to identify a country's HNP sector problems and achievements through comparisons with regional and income group aggregates. The World Bank is now starting to use this information to produce country-specific "*HNP At-A-Glance*" reports. These briefs disclose countries that are at greatest risk for poor HNP outcomes and help identify emerging issues to those charged with formulating country assistance strategies. The data collection effort that took place in preparing the *HNP Sector Strategy* has boosted the ability to monitor sectoral performance at the country level and to analyze the comparative success of the Bank's efforts across countries.

Data Sources and Limitations

The data presented in the tables can be divided into two broad groups: 1) those that have been analyzed and, where necessary, adjusted by the Bank's HNP staff, and 2) those obtained from other departments in the Bank, UN agencies, or other sources, and have not been separately analyzed for accuracy and consistency.

The *HNP Sector Strategy* focused on trends in health status, especially mortality indicators, and on health finance indicators, both of which fall in the first group of data. Disease-specific indicators, nutrition indicators, burden of disease estimates, and indicators of the determinants of health are generally obtained from other sources. For these indicators, UN and other agencies with specialized expertise are able to provide data that can give a more complete picture of the HNP situation of each country. For a few other indicators, that is, maternal mortality ratios or health services data, existing sources have been used (mainly WHO and official government data) with updates inserted where available.

Demographic indicators and vital rates were gathered from national statistical offices, the UN Statistical Office and Population Division, household surveys, and censuses. Current estimates of population and vital rates are examined annually by the Bank's country departments, and thus reflect the most recent information available. In many cases, however, the absence of population registers or vital registration make it inevitable that current estimates of many demographic indicators are projections based on indicators collected at the latest census or survey. Detailed information on the date of the most recent census, the latest demographic or household survey, and the completeness of vital registration can be found in *World Development Indicators 1998* (see bibliography).

The health finance indicators in the tables are the product of an extensive Bank effort, undertaken as part of the HNP sector strategy, to collect all such available information from household surveys, insurance publications, national accounts, local and central budgets, international donors, and existing tabulations. Such tabulations are published or made available by the International Monetary Fund (IMF), Pan American Health Organization (PAHO), Organization for Economic Cooperation and Development (OECD), and the World Bank in its public expenditure reviews and country and sector reports. Efforts to compile comprehensive cross-country data on health expenditures date back to the 1960s for Western Europe and North America (see Abel-Smith 1963, 1967.) The OECD started to compile such information for its member countries in 1977, leading to the development of a system of national health accounts that is only now beginning to be used in some developing countries. The World Bank's *World Development Report 1993: Investing in Health* was the first major effort to compile health expenditures for all developing countries. The health finance tables in this handbook are essentially an expanded update of that 1993 work.

Despite these efforts, cross-country comparisons of health financing data are often difficult because of the lack of reliable data on out-of-pocket expenditures. Where these exist at all, estimates are often incomplete and prone to measurement errors. Furthermore, private health expenditures are rarely disaggregated into different forms of payments, such as direct fees for service, insurance premiums or other forms of prepayments, and cost-sharing payments. Although efforts have been made to ensure comparability across countries, all findings should be interpreted with caution.

Health services availability and health services utilization indicators are also based on a comprehensive effort undertaken as part of the HNP sector strategy. Many countries lack data on the total number of health personnel, and others incorrectly include retired physicians or those working outside the health sector. The definition of nurses varies extensively among developing countries and cross-country comparability would be misleading; thus no indicator on the number of nurses has been included.

Health status, health finance, and health services indicators are presented as national averages, which conceal large differences among urban and rural areas as well as between geographical areas within countries. For operational purposes, further breakdowns would be essential for focusing interventions.

Definitions and sources of each of the indicators used in this statistical handbook follow the main tables.

Despite efforts to produce valid and comparable statistics, considerable uncertainty regarding the reliability of the data remains for many indicators and countries. This is a concern not only for health finance or health services indicators, as discussed above, but for even the most basic demographic data. Population censuses, for example, tend to be conducted only once every ten years in most countries (a few countries have censuses five years apart), involve long processing times, and are often not analyzed with sufficient attention to data quality. Government commitment to data collection, including allocation of sufficient human and financial resources, is lacking in many countries (see World Bank 1997, 1998). United Nations agencies that have been mandated with standardizing concepts and collecting comparative statistics are underfinanced, resulting in long delays in the dissemination of results. United Nations publications in demography, for example, often do not reflect the latest population census or demographic and health surveys. Other health indicators may be distorted, exagerrated, or otherwise misused by special interest groups to advocate one issue or disease over others, casting doubt on the validity and internal consistency of the data for all diseases.

Few would disagree that good policies need to be based on reliable data. But the limited data collection capacity of many borrowing countries, coupled with a relative lack of emphasis on improving statistical systems on the part of the World Bank and its partners, has led to decisionmaking—by the Bank as well as its borrowers—that is rarely based on sound empirical data.

What can the Bank do? The need to improve the monitoring and evaluation of projects and development outcomes is already being addressed in the Bank's country and sector strategies. Policy dialogue could further stress the importance of establishing health information systems that can meet the needs for project design and outcome evaluation. Investing in the development of data-gathering capability would be a logical next step.

Statistical Methods

Aggregates shown at the bottom of the tables in this handbook are based on the available data; that is, missing cases are excluded and no imputation was done. No aggregates are shown when data are missing for more than 50 percent of population-weighted cases in a particular region or income aggregate.

Total health expenditures are shown in real per capita terms in 1994 US dollars and in purchasing power parity (PPP) dollars. Public, private, and total health expenditures are shown as a percentage of GDP, and the public sector is also shown as a share of total health expenditures. Health expenditure aggregates shown in the tables are weighted by the population of the countries included in the aggregate.

In addition to weighting by population, health expenditure aggregates may be unweighted (that is, country-weighted, with each country having the same weight), or weighted by income. Table A compares the unweighted, population-weighted, and income-weighted averages for the world by income groups and also by Bank regions. In most regions income-weighted aggregate health expenditures are higher than population-weighted aggregate health expenditures. This indicates that countries with higher incomes spend more on health than countries with lower incomes. The greatest discrepancy between income- and population-weighted averages occurs in Sub-Saharan Africa. There, the income-weighted average is skewed toward South Africa, which exceeds two-thirds of the income for the region, whereas the population-weighted average is heavily

Table A. Health Expenditures by Income Group and Region

| | Health expenditure as % of GDP | | | | | | | | | Public share of health expenditure | | |
Region or income group	Total weighted average By income	By population	Total unweighted average	Public weighted average By income	By population	Public unweighted average	Private weighted average By income	By population	Private unweighted average	Weighted average By income	By population	Unweighted average
World	9.2	5.4	5.6	5.5	3.2	3.5	3.6	2.8	2.3	61	49	57
Low-income	4.2	4.2	4.0	1.6	1.5	2.1	2.6	2.7	2.2	39	37	49
Excl. China and India	3.1	3.1	4.0	1.2	1.1	2.1	2.0	2.0	2.2	36	37	50
Middle-income	5.9	5.1	5.8	3.2	4.3	4.0	3.0	2.4	2.5	51	52	56
Low- and middle-income	5.4	4.5	5.1	2.8	2.4	3.2	2.8	2.6	2.4	49	42	54
East Asia and Pacific	3.5	3.6	4.0	1.5	1.7	3.9	1.9	1.9	2.1	46	51	51
Europe and Central Asia	5.5	5.4	7.2	4.6	4.4	4.7	1.0	1.1	1.9	81	73	73
Latin America and Caribbean	7.2	6.7	6.1	3.0	2.9	3.2	4.2	3.9	2.9	41	49	49
Middle East and North Africa	4.0	4.5	5.1	2.6	2.4	2.6	2.2	2.2	2.6	54	50	50
South Asia	5.0	5.0	3.7	1.2	1.2	1.8	3.8	3.8	2.5	23	38	38
Sub-Saharan Africa	5.3	2.9	3.7	2.4	1.6	2.2	2.9	1.6	1.8	46	55	55
High-income	9.9	9.6	6.8	6.1	6.9	4.8	3.7	3.7	2.3	62	62	67
China			3.8			2.1			1.8	54	54	54
India			5.6			1.2			4.4	22	22	22
Established market econ.	10.1	10.1	8.1	6.4	6.4	6.1	3.8	3.7	2.0	62	62	67

influenced by Nigeria, with almost 20 percent of the region's population.

Regional and income aggregates for most other indicators are population-weighted averages. The weights are chosen to reflect the populations at risk. Aggregated infant mortality rates are weighted by the number of births in each country, child immunization is weighted by the population under age one, and life expectancies are weighted by the mortality schedules and population in each age group.

Population growth rates are shown as exponential growth rates between two points. This is calculated as:

$$\ln(p2/p1)/n$$

in which $p2$ and $p1$ are the last and first observation in the period, n is the number of years in the period, and ln is the natural logarithm. This growth rate is based on a model of continuous, exponential growth between two points in time. It does not take into account intermediate values. Population projections of the aging population and those underlying the burden of disease forecasts for 2020 are made using cohort component methods, in which the age-specific fertility, mortality, and migration rates are applied to the current age structure to obtain future populations.

Main Findings

The main output of the HNP indicator work consists of a set of tables showing country-level data as well as regional and income-group aggregates. These tables begin on page 19. This section highlights some of the main findings of these tables in terms of levels of health expenditures, patterns of availability and use of health services, levels and trends in health status, and correlates of health status.

Levels of Health Expenditure

Globally, countries spend an average of 5.4 percent of GDP on health, or about US$500 per capita per year. In the poorest countries total health expenditures may be as low as $3 per capita per year, largely from private sources. Low-income countries on average spend about 4 percent of GDP on health, with all countries in this group spending less than a dollar a day per person on health. Middle-income countries spend an average of 5 percent of GDP on health, but range from just $17 per capita in Indonesia to $1340 per capita in Iran. High-income countries spend an average of about 10 percent of GDP, ranging from $360 per capita per year in the Netherlands Antilles to $3,667 in the United States. By Bank region, Sub-Saharan Africa spends the least on health (about 3 percent of GDP), whereas the highest-spending region is Latin America and the Caribbean, which spends about 7 percent of GDP. Table B summarizes health expenditures by region and income group.

As per capita income increases, the public share of health spending increases as well. The average percentage of public spending was 37 percent for low-income countries, 52 percent for middle-income countries, and 62 percent for high-income countries. As shown in table B and figures 1 and 2, there is considerable variation among countries and regions in the

Table B. Health Expenditures by Region and Income Group

Region or income group	Real per capita (1994 US$) GDP	Real per capita (1994 US$) Total health expenditure	Per capita (PPP $) GDP	Per capita (PPP $) Total health expenditure	Health expenditure % of GDP Total	Health expenditure % of GDP Public	Health expenditure % of GDP Private	Public sector (% of total)
World	5,718	505	6,373	532	5.4	3.2	2.8	48.5
Low-income	623	22	1,893	78	4.2	1.5	2.7	36.8
Excluding China and India	939	18	1,518	47	3.1	1.1	2.0	36.7
Middle-income	3,761	209	5,198	264	5.1	4.3	2.4	52.3
Low- and middle-income	1,654	83	3,027	139	4.5	2.4	2.6	42.3
East Asia and Pacific	753	27	3,023	106	3.6	1.7	1.9	50.7
Europe and Central Asia	2,464	138	4,331	315	5.4	4.4	1.1	72.8
Latin America and the Caribbean	3,435	248	6,153	425	6.7	2.9	3.9	49.0
Middle East and North Africa	9,336	433	4,888	211	4.5	2.4	2.2	49.6
South Asia	407	21	1,348	64	5.0	1.2	3.8	38.5
Sub-Saharan Africa	1,814	55	1,729	87	2.9	1.6	1.6	55.4
High-income	24,022	2,404	21,788	2,227	9.6	6.9	3.7	62.0

Figure 1. Per Capita Total Health Expenditure, PPP$

Log per capita total health expenditure (PCHEXP)

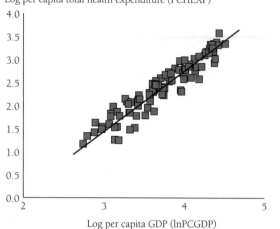

Log per capita GDP (lnPCGDP)

Note: lnPCHEXP = –2.19+1.24 lnPCGDP; Adjusted R^2 = 0.90; n = 102.

Figure 2. Per Capita Public Health Expenditure, PPP$

Log per capita public helath expenditure (PCPHEXP)

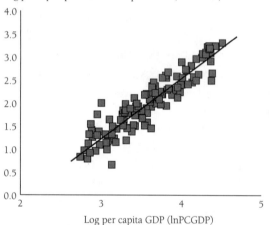

Log per capita GDP (lnPCGDP)

Note: lnPCPHEXP = –2.77+1.33 lnPCGDP; Adjusted R^2 = 0.88; n = 130.

proportion of health expenditure that is public. In South Asia less than 40 percent of spending on health is public, whereas the figure is more than 70 percent in Europe and Central Asia. Countries that have very low proportions of public health expenditures include India (22 percent), Vietnam (22 percent) and Nigeria (25 percent). Countries with very high proportions of public expenditures include Ghana (94 percent), Russia (87 percent), and Zambia (78 percent).

Income elasticities measure the percentage change in health expenditures as a result of changes in income. Globally, the income elasticity for health is estimated at 1.24, meaning that per capita health expenditures will increase by 1.24 percent for every 1 percent increase in per capita income. Income elasticity for public health

expenditures is estimated at 1.33: that is, for every 1 percent increase in per capita income, public health expenditure increases by 1.33 percent. The income elasticity for private health spending is estimated at 0.99, meaning that public health spending is more responsive to income changes than private health spending. Income elasticities for public health sector spending for income groups are shown in table C. Figures 3, 4, and 5 show the relationship between income and health spending within low-, middle-, and high-income groups.

Availability and Use of Health Services

The wide disparity in the number of doctors and beds per population across regions and income groups is shown in figures 6 and 7. Figure 6 shows the oversupply of physicians in the low- and middle-income countries of the Europe and Central Asia (ECA) region, where there are one-third more physicians than in the high-income countries. In Sub-Saharan Africa, in contrast, there is only one physician for every 10,000 people, creating an obstacle in the delivery of public health interventions and provision of a minimal package of essential clinical services (World Bank 1993). Figure 7 indicates an oversupply of hospital beds in the ECA region, which has more than 13 times the number of beds per 1,000 people than South Asia, the region with the lowest proportion of hospital beds per population.

Facilities and utilization of health services vary greatly across countries and even within regions and income groups. Figure 8 compares the number of outpatient visits to public providers for a number of countries. Figure 9 shows the average length of stay in public hospitals, and Figure 10 shows bed occupancy rates. The underutilization of public facilities in many countries is evident.

Table C. Income Eleasticity for Public Health Expenditure, by Income Group

Income group	Income elasticity	Number of observations	Adjusted R^2
Low-income	1.08	42	0.36
Middle-income	1.96	58	0.53
High-income	1.96	30	0.53
World	1.33	130	0.88

Figure 3. Income and Health Spending for Low-Income Countries, PPP$

Log per capita public health expenditure (lnPCPHEXP)

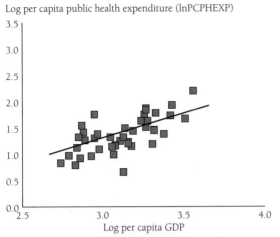

Note: lnGDP = −2.00+1.08 lnPCPHEXP; Adjusted R^2 = 0.43; n = 42.

Figure 4. Income and Health Spending for Middle-Income Countries, PPP$

Log per capita public health expenditure (lnPCPHEXP)

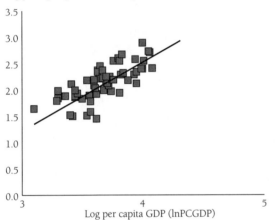

Note: lnPCPHEXP = −1.91+1.10 lnPCGDP; Adjusted R^2 = 0.53; n = 58.

Figure 5. Income and Health Spending for High-Income Countries, PPP$

Log per capita public health expenditure (lnPCPHEXP)

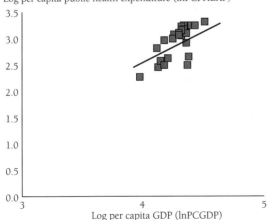

Note: lnPCPHEX = −5.46+1.96 lnGDP; Adjusted R^2 = 0.53; n = 30.

Figure 6. Inpatient Beds per 1,000 Population, by Income Group and Region

(*number of beds*)

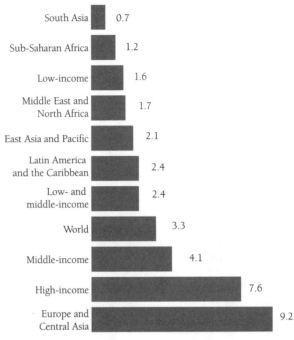

Figure 7. Doctors per 1,000 Population, by Income Group and Region

(*number of doctors*)

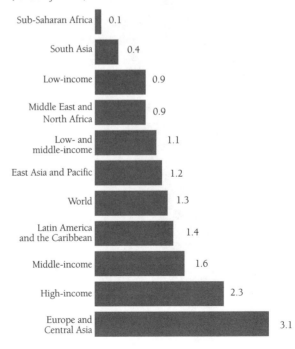

Figure 8. Outpatient Visits to Public Providers, Selected Countries

(visits per capita per year)

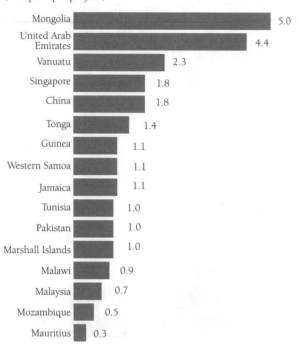

Mongolia	5.0
United Arab Emirates	4.4
Vanuatu	2.3
Singapore	1.8
China	1.8
Tonga	1.4
Guinea	1.1
Western Samoa	1.1
Jamaica	1.1
Tunisia	1.0
Pakistan	1.0
Marshall Islands	1.0
Malawi	0.9
Malaysia	0.7
Mozambique	0.5
Mauritius	0.3

Figure 9. Average Length of Stay in Public Hospital, Selected Countries

(days)

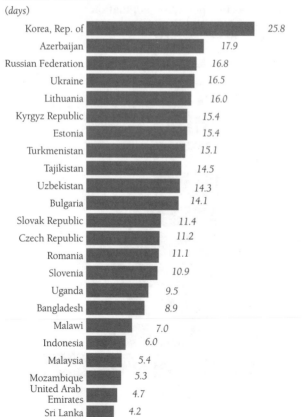

Korea, Rep. of	25.8
Azerbaijan	17.9
Russian Federation	16.8
Ukraine	16.5
Lithuania	16.0
Kyrgyz Republic	15.4
Estonia	15.4
Turkmenistan	15.1
Tajikistan	14.5
Uzbekistan	14.3
Bulgaria	14.1
Slovak Republic	11.4
Czech Republic	11.2
Romania	11.1
Slovenia	10.9
Uganda	9.5
Bangladesh	8.9
Malawi	7.0
Indonesia	6.0
Malaysia	5.4
Mozambique	5.3
United Arab Emirates	4.7
Sri Lanka	4.2

Figure 10. Bed Occupancy Rate in Public Hospitals, Selected Countries

(percent)

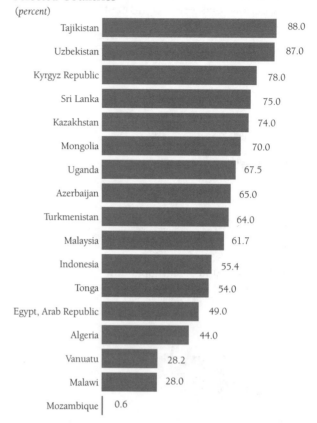

Tajikistan	88.0
Uzbekistan	87.0
Kyrgyz Republic	78.0
Sri Lanka	75.0
Kazakhstan	74.0
Mongolia	70.0
Uganda	67.5
Azerbaijan	65.0
Turkmenistan	64.0
Malaysia	61.7
Indonesia	55.4
Tonga	54.0
Egypt, Arab Republic	49.0
Algeria	44.0
Vanuatu	28.2
Malawi	28.0
Mozambique	0.6

Levels and Trends in Health Status

The tables provide convincing evidence of the substantial improvements in health outcomes occurring in most countries. Over the past 35 years, life expectancy has increased in virtually all countries, with infant and child mortality also improving substantially. Table D shows changes in life expectancy by region, and figure 11 shows trends in infant mortality rates for the world by region. Even in the Sub-Saharan African and South Asia regions, where health conditions are poorest, there have been large improvements in infant mortality rates and life expectancy.

These regional and income aggregates mask an important fact, however: while only a handful of countries have higher mortality now than in 1960, some countries have made much more progress than others. Moreover, there have been cases of reversals in the decline in mortality due to AIDS, chronic diseases, and regional conflicts. Figures 12 and 13 show trends in life expectancy in a number of countries, contrasting those

Table D. Life Expectancy at Birth, by Income Group and Region, 1960–95

Region or income group	1960	1970	1980	1990	1995
World	50	59	62	66	67
Low-income	40	54	58	61	63
Excluding China and India	42	46	51	53	56
Middle-income	55	59	64	67	68
Low- and middle-income	45	56	58	63	65
East Asia and Pacific	39	59	65	68	68
Europe and Central Asia	65	68	68	69	69
Latin America and the Caribbean	56	61	65	68	69
Middle East and North Africa	47	53	59	64	67
South Asia	44	49	54	59	62
Sub-Saharan Africa	41	44	48	51	52
High-income	70	71	74	76	78

Figure 11. Decline in Infant Mortality, by Region, 1960 and 1995

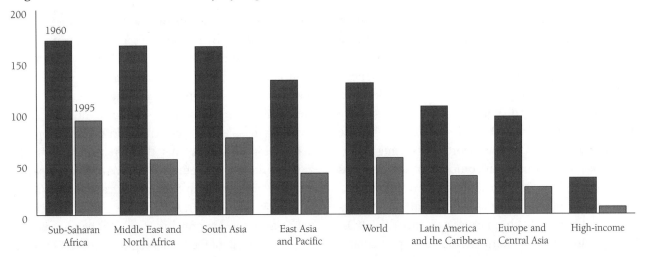

Figure 12. Mortality Decline in Six Countries that Have Made Little Progress: Trends in Live Expectancy, 1960–95

Life expectancy at birth (years)

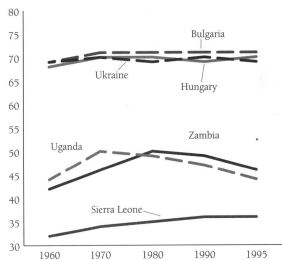

Figure 13. Mortality Decline in Six Countries that Have Made Good Progress: Trends in Live Expectancy, 1960–95

Life expectancy at birth (years)

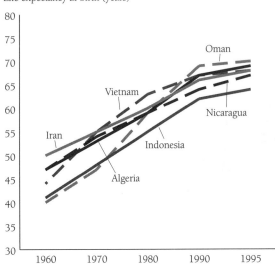

Figure 14. Adult Mortality, by Region, 1960–95

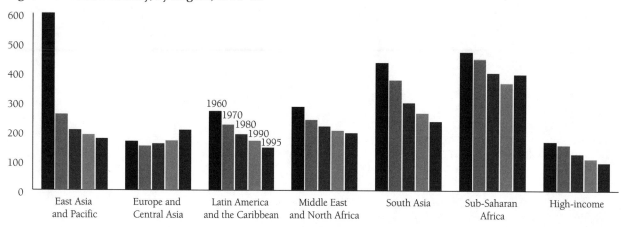

that have made a great deal of progress with those where life expectancy has increased much less or even recently declined.

Improvements in health status have not only been uneven across countries, but also across the life span. Generally, infant and child mortality rates have improved most, which is also reflected in increased life expectancy at birth. But adult mortality is rising in certain parts of the world. In some countries, this has occurred only since the mid-1980s, as a result of AIDS mortality; in other countries, adult male health has been declining due to chronic diseases since the 1960s. The increase in adult mortality has been particularly large in Russia and some of the other former Soviet republics. Figure 14 shows trends in adult male mor-

tality rates (shown as the probability of dying between ages 15 and 60) by region, over a 35-year period.

Most countries and regions have substantially reduced morbidity and mortality from certain causes, but are making less progress in other areas. For example, while overall mortality in South and East Asian countries has declined greatly, child malnutrition and maternal health problems there remain among the worst in the world (figure 15). HIV/AIDS has impacted mortality mostly in Sub-Saharan Africa so far (figure 16) but is now spreading in Asia and the Latin America and the Caribbean region as well. Tuberculosis has reemerged in all of the Bank's regions (figure 17), while high fertility remains a source of poor maternal health in three regions (figure 18).

Figure 15. Child Malnutrition, by Region, 1985–95
Percentage of malnourished children

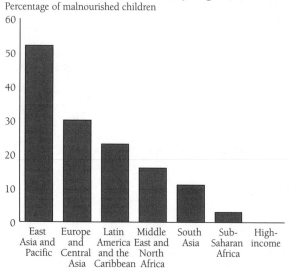

Figure 16. Adult HIV Prevalence, by Region, about 1995
Percentage HIV positive

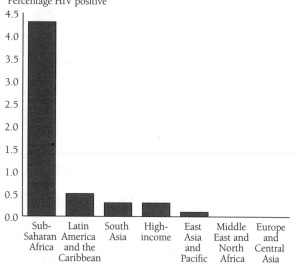

Figure 17. Tuberculosis Incidence, by Region, 1995

Smear positive incidence per 100,000 population

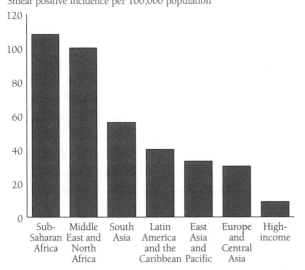

Figure 18. Fertility above Replacement Level, by Region, 1995

Total fertility rate above 2.1

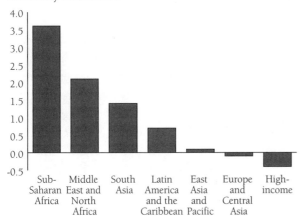

Projected changes in the age structure of populations will change disease patterns, causes of death, and the demand for health care. The number of people over age 60 is projected to increase in all of the Bank's regions, but especially in the Europe and Central Asia (ECA) and East Asia and Pacific (EAP) regions (figure 19). The composition of the burden of disease is projected to change not only because of demographic changes, but also because of the epidemiological transition that many low- and middle-income countries are currently experiencing. Changes in epidemiology are shifting the burden of disease from infectious and parasitic diseases to noncommunicable diseases and injuries. This trend is

Figure 19. Population over Age 60, by Region, 1990 and 2020

Percentage of total population over age 60

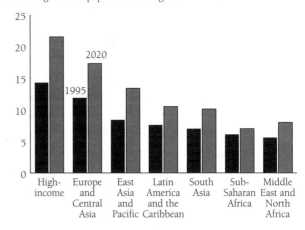

amplified by changes in age structure, as those age groups that are most subject to communicable diseases become a smaller proportion of the total, whereas the working-age adult populations and the elderly increase in number (figures 20, 21).

Figure 20. Global Burden of Disease, 1990

(*percent*)

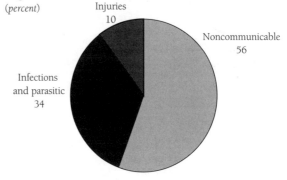

Figure 21. Global Burden of Disease, 2020

(*percent*)

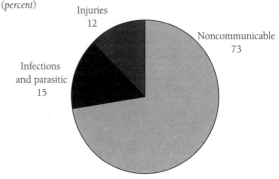

Correlates of Health Status

This section reviews the relationship between a number of socioeconomic indicators and health outcomes at the country and regional levels.

The importance of income as a determinant of health status is well established. In general, the poorer a country, the lower its population's life expectancy. This is illustrated in figure 22, which shows the estimated regression line between GNP per capita and life expectancy at birth in 1995. In addition to the strong relationship between life expectancy and per capita income, some countries (those far above the line) achieve considerably better life expectancy for a given level of income than other countries (those far below

the line). At a GNP per capita level of $600, for example, life expectancy in Honduras is 69 years (7 years better than predicted by the regression equation), whereas life expectancy in Senegal is only 51 years (11 years below the regression line). Thus while the relationship between income and health is strong, some countries have achieved healthy conditions at relatively low levels of income.

It is well known that people with more schooling enjoy better health (World Bank 1993). Even controlling for income, the relationship remains strong. Figure 23 shows the relationship between countries' average secondary school enrollment and under-five mortality rates. Similar associations exist for the impact of education on adult health.

A high degree of urbanization is associated with better health, both across countries and in comparisons of urban and rural populations within countries. Overall, urban populations tend to suffer less from infectious childhood diseases and child malnutrition, have lower fertility, and have better access to health services and sanitation. Urban incomes also tend to be higher, but the relationship holds even when GNP per capita is held constant. Figure 24 illustrates this relationship.

Other important determinants of health that are outside the direct control of the health sector are access to safe water and sanitation. Figures 25 and 26 show the relationships with life expectancy. In both cases, there is a significant relationship even when per capita GNP is held constant.

Figure 22. Income and Life Expectancy, All Countries, 1995 (*n=158*)

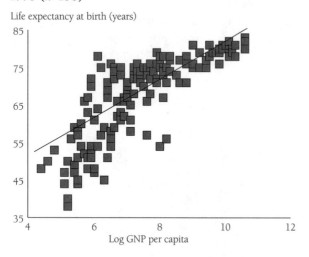

Life expectancy at birth (years)

Log GNP per capita

Figure 23. Secondary School Enrollment and Under-Five Mortality, All Countries, 1995 (*n=135*)

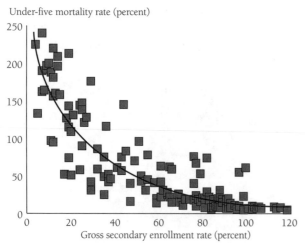

Under-five mortality rate (percent)

Gross secondary enrollment rate (percent)

Figure 24. Urbanization and Life Expectancy, All Countries, 1995 (*n=165*)

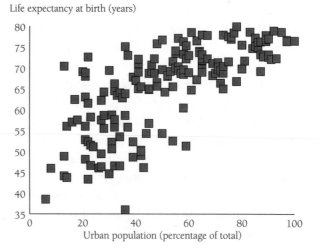

Life expectancy at birth (years)

Urban population (percentage of total)

Figure 25. Access to Safe Water and Life Expectancy, All Countries, 1990–95 (*n=93*)

Life expectancy at birth (years)

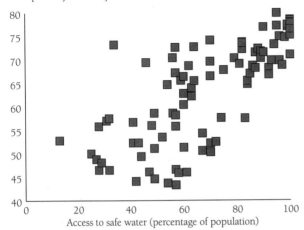

Access to safe water (percentage of population)

Figure 26. Access to Sanitation and Life Expectancy, All Countries, 1990–95 (*n=110*)

Life expectancy at birth (years)

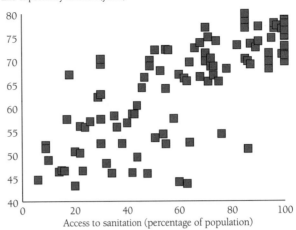

Access to sanitation (percentage of population)

Statistical Tables

Table 1. Health Expenditures, Basic Indicators

Economy	Year	Real per capita (1994 US$)		Per capita (1994 PPP $)		Health expenditure			
		GDP	Total health expenditure	GDP	Total health expenditure	Total[a]	Percent of GDP Public sector	Private sector	Public sector (% of total)
Afghanistan		..	..	..	..	..		..	..
Albania	1995	666	..	..	..	..	2.5	..	..
Algeria	1993	1,583	72	4,690	214	4.6	3.3	1.3	72.5
Angola	1991	534	..	2,302	..	..	4.1	..	..
Anguilla	1994	7,455	385	..	..	5.2	2.7	2.5	52.0
Antigua and Barbuda	1994	7,671	416	9,251	501	5.4	2.9	2.5	54.2
Argentina	1994	8,217	799	9,575	931	9.7	4.3	5.4	44.4
Armenia	1995	336	26	1,938	151	7.8	3.1	4.7	39.7
Aruba	1993	..	..	..	..	..		2.0	..
Australia	1996	19,147	1,653	19,775	1,707	8.6	5.7	2.9	66.5
Austria	1996	24,994	1,992	20,832	1,661	8.0	6.0	2.0	74.9
Azerbaijan	1995	446	27	1,455	89	6.1	1.1	5.0	18.5
Bahamas, The	1994	12,408	527	10,847	460	4.2	2.5	1.7	58.9
Bahrain	1990	7,746	538	13,631	947	7.0		..	..
Bangladesh	1995	224	5	936	23	2.4	1.2	1.3	48.1
Barbados	1994	6,541	448	10,224	700	6.8	4.4	2.4	64.7
Belarus	1995	1,966	125	4,098	261	6.4	5.3	1.1	82.9
Belgium	1996	23,349	1,840	21,308	1,679	7.9	6.9	1.0	87.7
Belize	1994	2,614	210	4,196	338	8.0	6.0	2.0	75.1
Benin	1994	281	..	1,157	..	..	1.7	..	..
Bermuda	1992	29,512	993	..	..	3.4	0.5	2.8	16.0
Bhutan	1995	416	..	..	..	..	2.3	..	..
Bolivia	1994	761	54	2,733	194	7.1	4.1	3.0	58.0
Bosnia and Herzegovina		..	..	..	..	..	..	..	..
Botswana	1991	2,966	86	7,243	209	2.9	1.6	1.3	54.6
Brazil	1994	3,542	163	5,730	264	4.6	1.8	2.8	40.0
Brunei	1994	..	..	..	..	..	2.2	..	..
Bulgaria	1992	1,137	78	4,460	307	6.9	5.5	1.4	79.6
Burkina Faso	1992	194	11	935	51	5.5	2.3	3.2	42.3
Burundi	1995	158	..	638	..	..	0.8	..	..
Cambodia	1994	247	18	..	..	7.2	0.7	6.5	9.7
Cameroon	1994	609	8	1,755	24	1.4	1.0	0.4	71.6
Canada	1996	18,782	1,724	21,228	1,948	9.2	6.6	2.6	71.4
Cape Verde	1994	936	..	1,882	..	..	3.4	..	..
Cayman Islands	1994	27,634	1,121	..	..	4.1	2.1	2.0	51.6
Central African Republic	1995	281	..	1,480	..	..	1.9	..	..
Chad	1995	134	5	870	33	3.7	3.7	0.1	97.5
Channel Islands		..	..	..	..	..		..	..
Chile	1994	3,728	231	9,907	613	6.2	2.5	3.7	40.2
China	1993	406	15	2,411	92	3.8	2.1	1.8	53.8
Colombia	1994	1,941	143	6,492	477	7.4	2.9	4.4	39.7
Comoros	1993	439	5	1,897	22	1.2	0.9	0.2	78.8
Congo, Dem. Rep.	1990	229	..	1,535	..	..	0.2	..	..
Congo, Rep.	1992	781	50	1,811	115	6.3	3.2	3.2	49.8
Costa Rica	1994	2,516	215	6,374	544	8.5	6.3	2.2	73.6
Côte d'Ivoire	1995	592	21	1,613	56	3.5	1.4	2.1	40.5
Croatia	1994	2,978	301	4,096	414	10.1	8.5	1.6	83.7
Cuba	1994	..	..	..	..	..	7.9	..	..
Cyprus	1993	9,529	434	17,643	804	4.6		..	..
Czech Republic	1995	3,696	338	9,912	906	9.1	7.4	1.8	80.5
Denmark	1996	29,099	1,863	21,795	1,396	6.4	5.1	1.3	79.4
Djibouti		..	..	..	..	..	..	..	..
Dominica	1994	3,006	188	4,273	268	6.3	4.0	2.3	63.2
Dominican Republic	1994	1,395	79	3,991	227	5.7	1.8	3.9	31.5
Ecuador	1994	1,481	78	4,908	259	5.3	2.0	3.2	38.6
Egypt, Arab Rep.	1995	..	..	..	..	3.7	1.6	2.1	43.2
El Salvador	1994	1,463	86	2,620	153	5.9	2.4	3.4	41.3
Equatorial Guinea	1990	231	15	1,237	78	6.3	5.2	1.2	81.3
Eritrea	1994	..	..	..	..	2.0	1.1	0.9	54.9
Estonia	1995	2,696	..	4,238	..	..	6.4	..	..
Ethiopia	1996	98	3	491	13	2.6	1.6	1.0	60.7
Fiji	1992	2,260	76	3,859	129	3.4	2.3	1.1	68.2
Finland	1996	20,555	1,534	18,074	1,349	7.5	5.6	1.9	74.5
France	1996	23,595	2,281	20,728	2,004	9.7	7.8	1.9	80.7
French Guiana	1991	11,813	..	..	..	..		2.7	..
French Polynesia		..	..	..	..	..		..	..
Gabon	1995	3,959	..	7,130	..	..	0.5	..	..
Gambia, The	1995	302	..	1,241	..	..	2.0	..	..
Georgia	1995	696	..	1,565	..	..	0.6	..	..
Germany	1996	..	..	..	..	10.5	8.2	2.3	78.3
Ghana	1995	316	5	1,716	25	1.5	1.4	0.1	93.5
Greece	1996	9,786	579	11,983	709	5.9	4.9	1.0	82.9
Grenada	1994	2,879	150	4,455	232	5.2	2.8	2.4	53.3
Guadeloupe	1993	8,018	..	..	..	..		2.4	..
Guam		..	..	..	..	..		..	..

Table 1. Health Expenditures, Basic Indicators (*continued*)

Economy	Year	Real per capita (1994 US$) GDP	Real per capita (1994 US$) Total health expenditure	Per capita (1994 PPP $) GDP	Per capita (1994 PPP $) Total health expenditure	Health expenditure Percent of GDP Total[a]	Health expenditure Percent of GDP Public sector	Health expenditure Percent of GDP Private sector	Public sector (% of total)
Guatemala	1994	1,258	41	3,405	111	3.2	1.7	1.5	53.8
Guinea	1994	528	..	1,655	..	..	1.2	..	..
Guinea-Bissau	1994	226	..	950	..	..	1.1	..	..
Guyana	1994	657	34	2,370	123	5.2	4.3	0.9	82.9
Haiti	1990	359	11	1,607	49	3.6	1.3	2.3	39.5
Honduras	1991	587	33	2,027	113	5.6	2.8	2.8	50.0
Hong Kong, China	1994	21,672	948	22,200	971	4.4	1.9	2.5	43.6
Hungary	1994	4,045	295	6,448	470	7.3	6.8	0.5	93.2
Iceland	1996	24,583	1,968	21,286	1,704	8.0	6.7	1.3	83.5
India	1991	295	17	1,234	69	5.6	1.2	4.4	21.7
Indonesia	1994	927	17	2,950	54	1.8	0.6	1.1	36.7
Iran, Islamic Rep.	1990	1,121	54	4,788	230	4.8	2.8	2.0	58.0
Iraq		..	..	..	..	..	..	..	..
Ireland	1995	16,649	1,058	17,126	1,088	6.4	5.1	1.2	80.8
Israel	1993	13,943	578	16,029	664	4.1	..	..	..
Italy	1996	18,381	1,391	19,330	1,463	7.6	5.3	2.3	69.9
Jamaica	1994	1,566	76	3,612	176	4.9	2.5	2.4	51.2
Japan	1995	37,981	2,732	21,520	1,548	7.2	5.6	1.6	78.4
Jordan	1994	1,481	117	3,299	261	7.9	3.7	4.2	46.7
Kazakhstan	1994	1,172	..	3,314	..	..	2.2	..	..
Kenya	1992	268	7	1,086	28	2.6	1.6	1.0	61.6
Kiribati	1991	507	..	..	..	..	22.8[b]	..	..
Korea, Dem. Rep.		..	..	..	..	..	..	..	..
Korea, Rep.	1992	7,589	408	9,878	531	5.4	1.8	3.6	33.5
Kuwait	1994	16,463	..	26,001	..	..	3.6	..	..
Kyrgyz Republic	1995	316	..	1,904	..	..	3.5	..	..
Lao PDR	1995	359	9	1,147	30	2.6	1.3	1.3	48.3
Latvia	1995	2,165	..	3,395	..	..	4.4	..	..
Lebanon	1992	2,085	111	4,645	248	5.3	2.1	3.3	38.9
Lesotho	1994	395	..	1,432	..	..	4.1	..	..
Liberia		..	..	..	..	..	..	..	..
Libya		..	..	..	..	..	..	..	..
Lithuania	1995	2,083	..	4,111	..	..	4.8	..	..
Luxembourg	1995	37,455	2,620	30,215	2,113	7.0	6.5	0.5	92.8
Macao		..	..	..	..	..	..	..	..
Macedonia, FYR	1995	..	..	..	..	8.3	7.3	0.9	88.7
Madagascar	1995	228	..	907	..	..	1.1	..	..
Malawi	1995	150	..	596	..	..	2.3	..	..
Malaysia	1993	3,369	83	8,701	215	2.5	1.5	1.0	59.9
Maldives	1990	865	..	2,619	..	..	4.9	..	..
Mali	1991	197	5	672	18	2.7	1.2	1.5	45.9
Malta	1991	7,160	532	10,954	814	7.4	..	..	..
Marshall Islands	1993	..	..	..	..	..	12.4	..	..
Martinique	1992	11,308	..	..	..	..	..	..	..
Mauritania	1991	444	23	1,696	88	5.2	1.1	4.1	21.4
Mauritius	1993	3,072	122	7,836	311	4.0	2.3	1.7	58.3
Mayotte		..	..	..	..	..	..	..	..
Mexico	1995	4,308	182	7,370	311	4.2	2.4	1.9	56.0
Micronesia, Fed. Sts.		..	..	..	..	..	..	..	..
Moldova	1995	..	..	..	..	..	4.9	..	..
Mongolia	1992	298	14	1,790	85	4.7	4.4	0.4	92.0
Montserrat	1994	4,982	280	..	..	5.6	3.5	2.1	62.5
Morocco	1993	1,070	37	3,016	103	3.4	1.6	1.7	48.0
Mozambique	1991	76	..	482	..	..	4.6	..	..
Myanmar	1994	1,786	..	..	..	..	0.4	..	..
Namibia	1993	1,971	141	4,684	335	7.2	3.7	3.5	51.6
Nepal	1995	195	10	1,006	50	5.0	1.2	3.8	24.4
Netherlands	1996	22,771	1,948	19,698	1,685	8.6	6.6	2.0	77.0
Netherlands Antilles	1992	8,176	389	..	..	4.8	2.5	2.2	53.3
New Caledonia		..	..	..	..	..	..	..	..
New Zealand	1996	14,738	1,058	17,105	1,228	7.2	5.5	1.7	75.9
Nicaragua	1994	431	37	2,016	174	8.6	5.3	3.4	61.0
Niger	1995	178	..	903	..	..	1.6	..	..
Nigeria	1994	232	3	863	11	1.3	0.3	1.0	25.1
Norway	1996	30,478	2,396	22,529	1,771	7.9	6.5	1.4	82.5
Oman	1991	5,422	..	9,934	..	..	2.5	..	..
Pakistan	1991	394	14	1,413	49	3.5	0.8	2.7	22.0
Panama	1994	2,991	199	6,860	457	6.7	4.7	2.0	70.1
Papua New Guinea	1994	1,312	..	3,071	..	..	2.8	..	..
Paraguay	1994	1,667	86	3,375	173	5.1	1.8	3.3	35.8
Peru	1994	2,150	80	4,181	156	3.7	2.2	1.5	59.7
Philippines	1991	936	22	3,106	74	2.4	1.3	1.0	56.0
Poland	1992	2,233	135	4,726	286	6.0	5.0	1.1	82.5
Portugal	1996	8,963	738	12,992	1,069	8.2	4.9	3.3	59.8
Puerto Rico	1994	11,493	..	..	..	..	..	6.0	..

Table 1. Health Expenditures, Basic Indicators (*continued*)

Economy	Year	Real per capita (1994 US$)		Per capita (1994 PPP $)		Health expenditure			
						Percent of GDP			Public sector
		GDP	Total health expenditure	GDP	Total health expenditure	Total[a]	Public sector	Private sector	(% of total)
Qatar	1993	..	..	..	..	2.8	..	..	..
Reunion		..	..	..	..	..	..	..	..
Romania	1995	1,421	..	4,269	..	..	3.6	..	..
Russian Federation	1994	2,197	105	4,502	215	4.8	4.1	0.6	86.5
Rwanda	1990	221	..	896	..	..	1.9	..	..
Samoa	1992	855	..	..	..	..	3.1	..	..
São Tomé and Principe	1995	383	..	..	..	..	6.2	..	..
Saudi Arabia	1991	..	..	..	..	3.1	..	..	..
Senegal	1994	479	..	1,557	..	..	2.5	..	..
Seychelles	1994	6,595	..	..	..	..	4.0	..	..
Sierra Leone	1991	241	9	640	23	3.6	1.5	2.0	42.7
Singapore	1995	25,872	916	24,415	864	3.5	1.3	2.2	36.8
Slovak Republic	1992	2,564	..	6,246	..	..	4.6	..	..
Slovenia	1992	..	..	..	..	..	7.3	..	..
Solomon Islands	1991	795	44	2,109	117	5.6	4.8	0.8	85.6
Somalia		..	..	..	..	..	..	..	..
South Africa	1993	3,306	260	7,029	552	7.9	3.6	4.3	45.2
Spain	1996	12,922	1,000	14,881	1,151	7.7	5.9	1.8	76.3
Sri Lanka	1993	630	12	2,055	39	1.9	1.4	0.4	76.3
St. Kitts and Nevis	1994	5,415	285	6,692	352	5.3	3.2	2.0	61.2
St. Lucia	1994	3,358	128	4,827	185	3.8	2.5	1.3	66.1
St. Vincent and the Grenadines	1994	2,169	153	3,887	273	7.0	5.2	1.9	73.5
Sudan	1991	..	..	..	..	0.3	..	..	..
Suriname	1994	719	29	2,246	90	4.0	2.0	2.0	50.4
Swaziland	1995	1,170	..	3,205	..	..	2.8	..	..
Sweden	1996	23,497	1,722	18,802	1,378	7.3	5.9	1.5	80.2
Switzerland	1995	37,384	3,651	24,124	2,356	9.8	7.0	2.7	71.9
Syrian Arab Republic		..	..	..	..	..	..	..	..
Taiwan, China	1993	10,871	530	14,888	726	4.9	2.6	2.3	53.6
Tajikistan	1994	386	..	1,127	..	..	5.8	..	..
Tanzania	1995	..	..	..	..	..	2.5	..	..
Thailand	1992	2,117	111	5,063	266	5.3	1.4	3.9	25.9
Togo	1991	288	10	1,873	64	3.4	1.2	2.2	35.1
Tonga	1992	1,500	..	..	..	..	4.0	..	..
Trinidad and Tobago	1994	3,838	131	6,167	211	3.4	2.1	1.3	60.8
Tunisia	1993	1,746	102	4,517	265	5.9	3.0	2.8	51.5
Turkey	1994	2,157	91	5,204	220	4.2	2.7	1.5	65.0
Turkmenistan	1994	993	..	2,260	..	..	1.2	..	..
Turks and Caicos Islands	1994	6,407	307	..	..	4.8	2.6	2.2	53.5
Uganda	1994	215	8	873	34	3.9	1.8	2.1	45.0
Ukraine	1995	891	..	2,370	..	..	4.9	..	..
United Arab Emirates	1994	15,178	379	15,599	390	2.5	2.0	0.5	81.1
United Kingdom	1996	18,136	1,254	19,104	1,321	6.9	5.8	1.1	84.3
United States	1996	26,539	3,723	26,907	3,775	14.0	6.6	7.4	47.0
Uruguay	1994	5,131	690	7,269	977	13.4	7.0	6.5	51.8
Uzbekistan	1994	942	..	2,470	..	..	3.5	..	..
Vanuatu	1993	1,109	..	2,739	..	..	3.3	..	..
Venezuela	1994	2,719	205	8,199	617	7.5	3.0	4.5	39.6
Vietnam	1993	201	11	1,229	64	5.2	1.1	4.1	21.7
Virgin Islands (UK)	1994	17,659	786	..	..	4.5	2.0	2.5	44.6
Virgin Islands (US)		..	..	..	..	..	..	..	..
West Bank and Gaza	1995	..	..	..	..	7.0	3.2	3.8	45.9
Yemen, Rep.	1994	407	10	734	19	2.5	1.1	1.4	43.5
Yugoslavia, Fed. Rep.		..	..	..	..	..	..	..	..
Zambia	1990	425	14	1,037	34	3.3	2.6	0.7	78.0
Zimbabwe	1991	582	36	2,351	145	6.2	2.2	4.0	35.1
World		4,598	438	5,743	476	5.3	2.6	2.7	48.2
Low-income		359	14	1,689	71	4.2	1.6	2.6	40.2
Excluding China and India		359	9	1,152	38	3.1	1.3	2.0	40.2
Middle-income		2,312	126	4,895	254	4.6	2.7	2.1	53.4
Lower middle		1,480	70	3,952	186	4.1	2.6	1.8	54.0
Upper middle		4,149	234	6,986	388	5.5	3.0	2.7	52.1
Low- and middle-income		1,002	50	2,715	130	4.3	1.9	2.5	44.4
East Asia and Pacific		612	20	2,620	93	3.6	1.7	1.9	49.3
Europe and Central Asia		1,848	121	4,185	261	5.3	4.1	1.1	79.1
Latin America and the Caribbean		3,534	202	6,230	356	5.5	2.6	3.0	46.0
Middle East and North Africa		1,640	61	4,209	172	4.3	2.3	2.1	51.9
South Asia		301	15	1,229	61	5.0	1.2	3.8	25.4
Sub-Saharan Africa		517	34	1,567	83	2.9	1.6	1.6	47.2
Excluding South Africa		295	8	1,132	30	2.3	1.5	1.3	47.4
High-income		23,647	2,339	21,365	2,170	9.6	6.0	3.6	65.3

Note: Averages in columns may not correspond because of differences in coverage of data.
a. Regional averages do not add up due to incomplete coverage of data for private health expenditures.
b. Includes foreign assistance totaling 12.5% of GDP for construction of new hospital.

Table 2. Health Expenditures, 1990–96

Economy	Total 1990	1991	1992	1993	1994	1995	1996	Public sector 1990	1991	1992	1993	1994	1995	1996	Private sector 1990	1991	1992	1993	1994	1995	1996
Afghanistan	..	..	..	..	..	..	..	..	..	..	..	..	..	..	..	..	..	..	..	..	..
Albania	..	..	..	..	..	..	..	3.3	4.4	3.0	2.7	2.5	2.5	..	..	..	..	..	..	..	..
Algeria	4.2	..	..	4.6	..	..	..	3.0	..	..	3.3	..	..	..	1.2	..	..	1.3	..	..	..
Angola	..	..	..	..	..	..	..	1.4	4.1	..	..	..	..	..	..	..	..	..	..	..	..
Anguilla	5.0	4.9	5.4	5.4	5.2	..	..	2.7	2.7	2.9	2.9	2.7	2.7	..	2.2	2.2	2.5	2.5	2.5	..	..
Antigua and Barbuda	4.9	4.9	4.9	4.9	5.4	..	..	2.8	2.8	2.8	2.8	2.9	3.7	..	2.1	2.1	2.1	2.1	2.5	..	..
Argentina	10.1	10.6	10.6	10.5	9.7	..	..	4.2	4.2	4.2	4.2	4.3	..	..	6.3	6.4	6.4	6.3	5.4	..	..
Armenia	..	..	..	..	..	7.8	..	..	..	4.7	3.6	1.5	3.1	..	..	..	..	..	..	4.7	..
Aruba	..	..	..	..	..	..	..	..	..	..	..	..	..	..	..	..	..	..	2.0	..	..
Australia	8.2	8.6	8.6	8.8	8.7	8.9	8.6	5.6	5.8	5.8	5.9	5.9	5.9	5.7	2.6	2.8	2.8	2.8	2.7	3.0	2.9
Austria	7.1	7.1	7.5	7.9	7.9	8.0	8.0	5.3	5.3	5.6	6.0	6.0	6.0	6.0	1.8	1.8	1.9	1.9	1.9	1.9	2.0
Azerbaijan	..	..	..	..	..	6.1	..	2.6	3.1	2.4	3.0	1.9	1.1	..	..	..	..	..	..	5.0	..
Bahamas, The	4.5	4.5	4.4	4.3	4.2	..	..	2.7	2.7	2.7	2.6	2.5	..	..	1.8	1.8	1.7	1.7	1.7	..	..
Bahrain	7.0	..	..	..	..	..	..	..	..	..	..	..	..	..	..	..	..	..	..	..	..
Bangladesh	..	..	..	..	..	2.4	..	1.1	1.0	1.0	1.2	1.2	1.2	..	..	..	..	..	..	1.3	..
Barbados	6.4	7.0	6.7	6.8	6.8	..	..	3.9	4.6	4.2	4.4	4.4	..	..	2.5	2.4	2.4	2.4	2.4	..	..
Belarus	..	..	..	..	..	6.4	..	2.6	3.1	3.4	4.7	5.2	5.3	..	..	..	..	..	..	1.1	..
Belgium	7.6	8.0	8.1	8.2	8.1	8.0	7.9	6.7	7.0	7.2	7.3	7.2	7.0	6.9	0.8	1.0	0.9	0.9	1.0	1.0	1.0
Belize	4.5	4.5	4.4	5.8	8.0	..	..	2.2	2.2	2.1	3.6	6.0	..	..	2.3	2.3	2.3	2.2	2.0	..	..
Benin	..	..	..	..	..	..	..	0.5	..	..	..	1.7	..	..	..	..	..	..	..	..	..
Bermuda	3.4	3.4	3.4	..	..	..	..	0.5	0.5	0.5	..	..	..	..	2.8	2.8	2.8	4.0	4.0	..	..
Bhutan	..	..	..	..	..	..	..	2.1	1.9	1.8	2.1	1.8	2.3	..	..	..	..	..	..	..	..
Bolivia	4.6	4.7	5.7	6.7	7.1	..	..	1.3	1.4	2.8	3.9	4.1	..	..	3.4	3.2	2.9	2.9	3.0	..	..
Bosnia and Herzegovina	..	..	..	..	..	..	..	..	..	..	..	..	..	..	..	..	..	..	..	..	..
Botswana	..	2.9	..	..	..	..	..	..	1.6	1.8	..	..	..	..	..	1.3	..	..	..	..	..
Brazil	6.8	6.6	6.5	6.7	4.6	..	..	2.9	2.0	1.7	2.1	1.8	..	..	3.9	4.7	4.8	4.6	2.8	..	..
Brunei	..	..	..	..	..	..	..	1.6	1.8	1.9	2.2	2.2	0.8	..	..	..	..	..	..	..	..
Bulgaria	5.2	5.2	6.9	..	..	..	..	4.1	4.4	5.5	4.9	4.2	3.8	..	1.1	0.9	1.4	..	..	..	..
Burkina Faso	..	..	5.5	..	..	..	..	..	..	2.3	..	..	..	..	..	1.1	3.2	..	..	..	..
Burundi	..	..	..	..	..	..	..	0.8	..	..	..	..	0.8	..	..	..	..	..	..	..	..
Cambodia	..	..	..	..	7.2	..	..	..	..	0.2	0.2	0.7	..	..	..	..	..	..	..	6.5	..
Cameroon	1.1	1.1	1.2	1.2	1.4	..	..	0.9	0.9	1.1	1.1	1.0	..	..	0.1	0.2	0.1	0.1	0.4	..	..
Canada	9.2	9.9	10.2	10.2	9.9	9.7	9.2	6.9	7.4	7.6	7.4	7.1	6.9	6.6	2.3	2.5	2.7	2.7	2.8	2.8	2.6
Cape Verde	..	..	..	..	..	..	..	..	3.2	2.6	3.2	3.4	3.3	..	..	..	..	..	..	..	..
Cayman Islands	4.2	4.0	4.7	4.0	4.1	..	..	2.3	2.0	2.8	2.1	2.1	2.4	..	1.9	2.0	1.9	2.0	2.0	..	..
Central African Republic	..	..	..	..	..	..	..	..	0.9	0.9	1.1	1.6	1.9	..	..	..	..	..	..	..	..
Chad	..	..	..	..	..	3.7	..	..	..	..	4.1	2.2	3.7	..	..	..	..	..	..	0.1	..
Channel Islands	..	..	..	..	..	..	..	..	..	..	..	..	..	..	..	..	..	..	..	..	..
Chile	6.2	6.3	6.3	6.4	6.2	..	..	2.0	2.2	2.3	2.4	2.5	2.3	..	4.3	4.2	4.1	4.0	3.7	..	..
China	3.5	3.5	3.4	3.8	..	..	..	2.1	2.1	2.0	2.1	..	..	..	1.3	1.5	1.4	1.8	..	..	..
Colombia	6.9	7.0	7.2	6.4	7.4	..	..	2.5	2.8	2.8	1.6	2.9	..	..	4.4	4.2	4.4	4.8	4.4	..	..
Comoros	..	..	..	1.2	..	..	..	..	..	..	0.9	0.8	1.0	..	..	..	..	..	0.2	..	..
Congo, Dem. Rep.	..	..	..	..	..	..	..	0.2	..	..	..	..	..	..	..	..	..	..	..	..	..
Congo, Rep.	2.6	..	6.3	..	..	..	..	1.5	..	3.2	2.4	1.8	..	..	1.1	..	3.2	..	..	..	..
Costa Rica	9.0	0.1	9.8	9.6	8.5	..	..	6.7	7.9	7.6	7.5	6.3	6.0	..	2.2	2.2	2.2	2.2	2.2	..	..
Côte d'Ivoire	..	..	..	..	..	3.5	..	..	1.6	1.7	1.6	1.6	1.4	..	..	..	..	..	..	2.1	..
Croatia	11.8	3.0	11.6	12.2	10.1	..	..	9.7	10.8	9.9	9.3	8.5	..	..	2.2	2.2	1.7	2.9	1.6	..	..
Cuba	..	..	..	..	..	..	..	4.6	5.2	6.2	8.1	7.9	..	..	..	..	..	..	..	..	..
Cyprus	..	4.3	..	4.6	..	..	..	..	..	..	..	..	..	..	..	..	..	..	..	..	..
Czech Republic	..	6.5	6.9	9.7	9.9	9.1	..	5.5	5.4	5.4	7.6	7.8	7.4	..	..	1.1	1.5	2.1	2.1	1.8	..
Denmark	6.5	6.5	6.6	6.8	6.6	6.4	6.4	5.3	5.5	5.6	5.6	5.5	5.3	5.1	1.1	1.1	1.1	1.1	1.1	1.1	1.3
Djibouti	..	..	..	..	..	..	..	..	..	..	..	..	..	..	..	..	..	..	..	..	..
Dominica	6.3	6.5	6.3	6.3	6.3	..	..	3.9	4.1	3.8	3.9	4.0	3.9	..	2.4	2.4	2.4	2.4	2.3	..	..
Dominican Republic	5.2	5.5	5.6	5.8	5.7	..	..	1.6	1.3	1.6	2.0	1.8	..	..	3.5	4.3	4.0	3.9	3.9	..	..
Ecuador	5.3	4.6	5.3	4.7	5.3	..	..	2.5	1.6	2.1	1.6	2.0	..	..	2.8	2.9	3.2	3.0	3.2	..	..
Egypt, Arab Rep.	4.3	..	..	..	..	3.7	..	1.8	..	..	..	..	1.6	..	2.5	..	..	..	..	2.1	..
El Salvador	5.1	5.2	5.2	5.0	5.9	..	..	1.4	1.5	1.6	1.1	2.4	..	..	3.7	3.7	3.6	3.9	3.4	..	..
Equatorial Guinea	6.3	..	..	..	..	..	..	5.2	..	..	..	..	..	..	1.2	..	..	..	..	..	..
Eritrea	..	..	..	..	2.0	..	..	..	..	0.6	0.8	1.1	..	..	..	..	..	..	..	0.9	..
Estonia	..	..	..	..	..	..	..	2.1	..	5.3	..	5.9	6.4	..	..	..	..	..	..	..	..
Ethiopia	..	..	..	..	..	..	2.6	1.0	0.8	0.9	1.0	1.8	1.7	1.6	..	..	..	..	..	..	1.0
Fiji	..	..	3.4	..	..	..	..	2.0	2.2	2.3	..	..	..	..	..	..	..	1.1	..	..	..
Finland	8.0	9.1	9.3	8.4	7.9	7.7	7.5	6.5	7.4	7.4	6.4	5.9	5.8	5.6	1.5	1.7	1.9	2.0	2.0	2.0	1.9
France	8.9	9.1	9.4	9.8	9.7	9.9	9.7	6.6	6.8	7.0	7.3	7.6	8.0	7.8	2.3	2.3	2.4	2.5	2.1	1.9	1.9
French Guiana	..	..	..	..	..	..	..	..	..	..	..	..	..	..	2.8	2.7	..	..	..	..	..
French Polynesia	..	..	..	..	..	..	..	..	..	..	..	..	..	..	..	..	..	..	..	..	..
Gabon	..	..	..	..	..	..	..	..	0.5	0.7	0.8	0.5	0.5	..	..	..	..	..	..	..	..
Gambia, The	..	..	..	..	..	..	..	2.3	1.9	1.9	1.8	2.0	..	..	..	..	..	..	..	..	..
Georgia	..	..	..	..	..	..	..	3.0	4.1	2.4	0.4	0.3	0.6	..	..	..	..	..	..	..	..
Germany	..	9.6	10.2	10.1	10.3	10.4	10.5	..	7.5	8.0	8.0	8.0	8.2	8.2	..	2.1	2.1	2.2	2.2	2.3	2.3
Ghana	..	..	..	..	1.1	1.5	..	1.5	..	..	..	1.1	1.4	..	..	..	..	..	0.1	0.1	0.1
Greece	4.2	4.2	4.5	5.0	5.5	5.8	5.9	3.5	3.4	3.4	3.8	4.2	4.4	4.9	0.7	0.8	1.1	1.2	1.3	1.4	1.0
Grenada	5.5	5.2	5.3	5.1	5.2	..	..	3.3	2.8	2.8	2.7	2.8	2.7	..	2.2	2.4	2.4	2.4	2.4	..	..
Guadeloupe	..	..	..	..	..	..	..	..	..	..	..	..	..	..	2.5	2.4	2.5	2.4	..	..	..
Guam	..	..	..	..	..	..	..	..	..	..	..	..	..	..	..	..	..	..	..	..	..

Table 2. Health Expenditures, 1990–96 (*continued*)

	Percent of GDP																				
	Total							Public sector							Private sector						
Economy	1990	1991	1992	1993	1994	1995	1996	1990	1991	1992	1993	1994	1995	1996	1990	1991	1992	1993	1994	1995	1996
Guatemala	3.0	2.9	3.0	3.1	3.2	..	..	1.5	1.4	1.4	1.6	1.7	..	..	1.5	1.6	1.6	1.5	1.5	..	..
Guinea	..	..	..	..	..	..	..	1.2	1.2	1.3	1.1	1.2	..	..	..	..	..	..	..	..	..
Guinea-Bissau	..	..	..	..	..	..	..	1.1	1.2	0.7	1.1	1.1	..	..	..	..	..	..	..	..	..
Guyana	3.8	3.1	4.8	5.1	5.2	..	..	2.9	2.1	3.9	4.2	4.3	..	..	0.9	1.0	0.9	0.9	0.9	..	..
Haiti	3.1	..	..	..	..	..	..	1.2	..	..	..	..	..	..	1.9	2.2	2.2	2.3	2.7	..	..
Honduras	4.9	5.6	..	..	..	..	..	2.1	2.8	..	..	..	..	..	2.8	2.8	2.8	2.8	2.8	..	..
Hong Kong, China	3.7	3.7	3.9	4.2	4.4	..	..	1.6	1.6	1.7	2.1	1.9	..	..	2.1	2.1	2.2	2.1	2.5	..	..
Hungary	5.9	7.0	7.0	7.3	7.3	..	..	5.7	6.7	6.6	6.8	6.8	..	..	0.2	0.3	0.4	0.4	0.5	..	..
Iceland	8.0	8.1	8.2	8.3	8.1	8.2	8.0	6.9	7.0	7.0	6.9	6.8	6.9	6.7	1.1	1.1	1.2	1.3	1.3	1.3	1.3
India	6.0	5.6	..	..	..	..	..	1.3	1.2	..	0.8	0.8	0.7	..	4.7	4.4	..	..	..	..	..
Indonesia	1.9	1.8	1.9	1.9	1.8	..	..	0.6	0.6	0.7	0.7	0.7	..	..	1.3	1.2	1.2	1.2	1.2	..	..
Iran, Islamic Rep.	4.8	..	..	..	..	..	..	2.8	..	1.0	1.0	1.3	1.3	..	2.0	..	..	..	..	..	..
Iraq	..	..	..	..	..	..	..	..	..	..	..	..	..	..	..	..	..	..	..	..	..
Ireland	6.6	6.8	7.1	7.1	7.6	6.4	..	4.9	5.3	5.5	6.3	6.1	5.1	6.0	1.7	1.6	1.6	0.8	1.5	1.2	..
Israel	4.2	..	..	4.1	..	..	..	2.1	..	..	..	..	..	..	2.1	..	..	..	..	..	..
Italy	8.1	8.4	8.5	8.6	8.4	7.7	7.6	6.3	6.6	6.5	6.3	5.9	5.4	5.3	1.8	1.8	2.0	2.3	2.5	2.4	2.3
Jamaica	4.0	3.4	3.5	5.2	4.9	..	..	2.6	2.3	2.3	3.0	2.5	..	..	1.3	1.1	1.2	2.3	2.4	..	..
Japan	6.1	6.1	6.3	6.6	6.9	7.2	..	4.7	4.8	4.9	5.2	5.3	5.6	..	1.4	1.3	1.4	1.4	1.6	1.6	..
Jordan	6.9	7.9	6.9	6.5	7.9	..	..	3.6	3.6	3.0	3.1	3.7	..	..	3.4	4.3	3.9	3.4	4.2	..	..
Kazakhstan	..	..	..	..	..	..	..	3.2	4.3	2.1	2.2	2.2	..	..	..	..	..	..	..	..	..
Kenya	..	..	2.6	..	..	..	..	1.7	1.7	1.6	1.9	..	..	..	..	..	1.0	..	..	..	..
Kiribati	..	..	..	..	..	..	..	8.3	22.8	..	..	..	..	..	..	..	..	..	..	..	..
Korea, Dem. Rep.	..	..	..	..	..	..	..	..	..	..	..	..	..	..	..	..	..	..	..	..	..
Korea, Rep.	5.1	4.9	5.4	..	..	..	..	1.9	1.7	1.8	..	..	..	..	3.2	3.2	3.6	..	..	..	..
Kuwait	..	..	..	..	..	..	..	4.0	1.9	3.8	3.3	3.6	..	..	..	..	..	..	..	..	..
Kyrgyz Republic	..	..	..	..	..	..	..	4.2	3.6	3.2	2.6	3.5	3.5	..	..	..	..	..	..	..	..
Lao PDR	..	..	..	4.9	..	2.6	..	1.0	..	..	3.1	..	1.3	..	..	..	..	1.8	..	1.3	..
Latvia	..	..	..	..	..	..	..	2.4	2.6	2.8	4.1	3.7	4.4	..	..	..	..	..	..	..	..
Lebanon	..	3.1	5.3	..	..	..	..	..	..	2.1	..	..	..	..	..	..	3.3	..	..	..	..
Lesotho	..	..	..	..	..	..	..	2.5	4.2	4.3	4.3	4.1	..	..	..	..	..	..	..	..	..
Liberia	..	..	..	..	..	..	..	..	..	..	..	..	..	..	..	..	..	..	..	..	..
Libya	..	..	..	..	..	..	..	..	..	..	..	..	..	..	..	..	..	..	..	..	..
Lithuania	..	..	..	..	..	..	..	3.1	3.3	3.8	3.9	4.8	4.8	..	..	..	..	..	..	..	..
Luxembourg	6.6	6.5	6.6	6.7	6.5	7.0	..	6.1	6.0	6.1	6.2	6.0	6.5	..	0.5	0.5	0.5	0.5	0.5	0.5	..
Macao	..	..	..	..	..	..	..	..	..	..	..	..	..	..	..	..	..	..	..	..	..
Macedonia, FYR	7.9	12.7	9.1	8.8	7.7	8.3	..	7.9	11.4	7.9	7.7	6.8	7.3	..	0.0	1.3	1.2	1.1	0.9	0.9	..
Madagascar	..	..	..	..	..	..	..	..	..	1.4	..	1.0	1.1	..	..	..	..	..	..	..	..
Malawi	..	..	..	..	..	..	..	..	..	..	..	..	2.3	..	..	..	..	..	..	..	..
Malaysia	..	..	..	2.5	..	..	..	1.5	1.6	1.6	1.5	1.4	..	..	..	..	..	..	1.0	..	..
Maldives	..	..	..	..	..	..	..	4.9	..	..	..	..	..	..	..	..	..	..	..	..	..
Mali	2.9	2.7	..	..	..	..	..	1.6	1.2	1.0	1.0	2.0	..	..	1.3	1.5	..	..	..	..	..
Malta	..	7.4	..	..	..	..	..	..	..	..	..	..	..	..	..	..	..	..	..	..	..
Marshall Islands	..	..	..	..	..	..	..	12.9	13.5	14.4	12.4	..	..	..	..	..	..	..	..	..	..
Martinique	..	..	..	..	..	..	..	..	..	..	..	..	..	..	2.8	2.6	2.9	..	..	..	..
Mauritania	..	5.2	..	..	..	..	..	..	..	1.1	1.1	1.2	1.5	1.8	..	4.1	..	..	..	..	..
Mauritius	..	3.4	3.6	4.0	..	..	..	..	2.1	2.3	2.3	2.2	..	..	..	1.3	1.3	1.7	..	..	..
Mayotte	..	..	..	..	..	..	..	..	..	..	..	..	..	..	..	..	..	..	..	..	..
Mexico	5.1	5.1	4.8	4.6	4.7	4.2	..	2.5	2.5	2.5	2.5	2.6	2.4	..	2.6	2.7	2.3	2.1	2.1	1.9	..
Micronesia, Fed. Sts.	..	..	..	..	..	..	..	..	..	..	..	..	..	..	..	..	..	..	..	..	..
Moldova	..	..	..	..	..	..	..	..	..	..	3.6	5.1	4.9	..	..	..	..	..	..	..	..
Mongolia	6.7	6.8	4.7	..	..	..	..	6.0	6.3	4.4	4.4	4.4	4.3	..	0.7	0.5	0.4	..	..	..	..
Montserrat	4.7	5.8	5.8	5.8	5.6	..	..	2.4	3.8	3.8	3.7	3.5	4.1	..	2.3	2.1	2.1	2.1	2.1	..	..
Morocco	2.5	3.1	..	3.4	..	..	..	0.9	..	..	1.6	..	..	..	1.6	..	..	1.7	..	..	..
Mozambique	..	..	..	..	..	..	..	4.4	4.6	..	..	..	..	..	..	..	..	..	..	..	..
Myanmar	..	..	..	..	..	..	..	1.0	1.0	0.8	0.5	0.4	..	..	..	..	..	..	..	..	..
Namibia	..	4.9	..	7.2	..	..	..	3.1	3.4	4.2	3.7	3.5	..	..	..	1.5	..	3.5	..	..	..
Nepal	..	..	..	..	..	5.0	..	1.0	..	0.5	..	..	1.2	..	..	..	..	..	..	3.8	..
Netherlands	8.3	8.6	8.8	8.9	8.8	8.8	8.6	6.1	6.4	6.8	7.0	6.8	6.8	6.6	2.3	2.2	2.0	1.9	2.0	2.0	2.0
Netherlands Antilles	4.0	4.2	4.8	..	..	..	..	1.6	1.9	2.5	..	..	..	..	2.4	2.3	2.2	..	..	..	..
New Caledonia	..	..	..	..	..	..	..	..	..	..	..	..	..	..	..	..	..	..	..	..	..
New Zealand	7.0	7.5	7.6	7.3	7.1	7.1	7.2	5.8	6.1	6.0	5.6	5.4	5.4	5.5	1.2	1.3	1.6	1.7	1.6	1.7	1.7
Nicaragua	8.1	7.6	8.0	8.1	8.6	..	..	4.8	3.8	4.0	3.9	5.3	..	..	3.3	3.8	4.0	4.2	3.4	..	..
Niger	..	..	..	..	..	..	..	..	1.5	1.6	1.7	2.1	1.6	..	..	..	..	..	..	..	..
Nigeria	..	..	..	..	1.3	..	..	1.0	0.9	1.1	0.8	0.3	..	..	..	..	..	..	1.0	..	..
Norway	7.8	8.1	8.2	8.1	8.0	8.0	7.9	6.5	6.8	7.0	6.7	6.7	6.6	6.5	1.3	1.3	1.2	1.3	1.4	1.4	1.4
Oman	..	..	..	..	..	..	..	2.0	2.5	..	..	..	..	..	..	..	..	..	..	..	..
Pakistan	..	3.5	..	..	..	..	..	0.8	0.8	0.8	0.8	0.8	0.8	..	..	2.7	..	..	..	..	..
Panama	7.2	7.8	6.6	6.7	6.7	..	..	5.3	6.0	4.7	4.9	4.7	..	..	1.9	1.8	1.9	1.8	2.0	..	..
Papua New Guinea	..	..	..	..	..	..	..	3.1	2.8	2.4	2.8	2.8	..	..	..	..	..	..	..	..	..
Paraguay	4.3	4.2	4.2	4.3	5.1	..	..	0.4	0.8	0.8	1.0	1.8	..	..	3.8	3.5	3.5	3.3	3.3	..	..
Peru	3.2	4.2	4.0	3.7	3.7	..	..	1.0	2.2	2.5	2.2	2.2	..	..	2.2	2.1	1.5	1.5	1.5	..	..
Philippines	..	2.4	..	..	..	..	..	0.8	1.3	..	..	..	..	..	..	1.0	..	..	..	..	..
Poland	5.1	5.8	6.0	..	..	..	..	4.8	5.1	5.0	4.6	4.6	4.8	..	0.3	0.7	1.1	..	..	..	..
Portugal	6.5	7.2	7.4	7.7	7.8	8.2	8.2	4.3	4.5	4.4	4.8	4.9	5.0	4.9	2.3	2.7	3.0	2.8	2.9	3.3	3.3
Puerto Rico	..	..	..	..	..	..	..	..	..	..	..	..	..	..	5.0	5.7	6.0	6.0	6.0	..	..

Table 2. Health Expenditures, 1990–96 (*continued*)

	Total							Public sector							Private sector						
											Percent of GDP										
Economy	1990	1991	1992	1993	1994	1995	1996	1990	1991	1992	1993	1994	1995	1996	1990	1991	1992	1993	1994	1995	1996
Qatar	..	3.2	..	2.8	..	..	..	..	..	..	..	..	..	..	..	..	..	..	..	..	..
Reunion	..	..	..	..	..	..	..	..	..	..	..	..	..	..	..	..	..	..	..	..	..
Romania	..	..	..	..	..	..	..	2.8	3.3	3.6	3.0	3.3	3.6	..	..	..	..	..	..	..	..
Russian Federation	..	2.6	2.6	3.5	4.8	..	..	2.5	2.4	2.5	3.3	4.1	..	..	..	0.2	0.1	0.2	0.6	..	..
Rwanda	..	..	..	..	..	..	..	1.9	..	..	..	..	..	..	..	..	..	..	..	..	..
Samoa	..	..	..	..	..	..	..	5.1	4.8	3.1	3.6	..	..	..	..	..	..	..	..	..	..
São Tomé and Principe	..	..	..	..	..	..	..	..	..	..	3.1	2.7	6.2	..	..	..	..	..	..	..	..
Saudi Arabia	..	2.2	..	..	..	..	..	..	..	..	..	..	3.1	..	..	..	..	..	..	..	..
Senegal	..	..	..	..	..	..	..	2.8	..	..	2.4	2.5	..	..	..	..	..	..	..	..	..
Seychelles	..	..	..	..	..	..	..	3.5	3.9	4.0	..	4.0	4.1	..	..	..	..	..	..	..	..
Sierra Leone	..	3.6	..	..	..	..	..	..	1.5	1.6	..	..	..	..	..	2.0	..	..	..	..	..
Singapore	3.3	3.4	3.4	3.5	3.4	3.5	..	1.1	1.1	1.1	1.0	1.1	1.3	..	2.2	2.2	2.2	2.5	2.3	2.2	..
Slovak Republic	..	..	..	..	..	..	..	5.0	4.6	4.6	..	..	..	..	..	..	..	..	..	..	..
Slovenia	..	..	..	..	..	..	..	7.1	5.2	7.3	..	..	..	..	..	..	..	..	..	..	..
Solomon Islands	..	5.6	..	..	..	..	..	..	4.8	..	..	..	..	..	..	0.8	..	..	..	..	..
Somalia	..	..	..	..	..	..	..	..	..	..	..	..	..	..	..	..	..	..	..	..	..
South Africa	..	..	..	7.9	..	..	..	..	..	..	3.6	..	..	..	..	..	..	4.3	..	..	..
Spain	6.9	7.1	7.2	7.3	7.3	7.6	7.7	5.4	5.6	5.7	5.7	5.7	6.0	5.9	1.5	1.5	1.5	1.6	1.6	1.7	1.8
Sri Lanka	..	..	..	1.9	..	..	..	1.7	1.5	1.6	1.4	1.4	..	..	..	..	..	..	0.4	..	..
St. Kitts and Nevis	4.9	4.9	4.9	5.1	5.3	..	..	2.7	2.7	2.7	2.9	3.2	3.1	..	2.2	2.1	2.2	2.1	2.0	..	..
St. Lucia	3.4	3.5	3.4	3.7	3.8	..	..	2.1	2.1	2.1	2.4	2.5	2.5	..	1.3	1.3	1.3	1.3	1.3	..	..
St. Vincent and the Grenadines	6.4	5.8	5.8	6.0	7.0	..	..	4.5	3.9	3.8	4.1	5.2	5.3	..	1.9	2.0	2.0	2.0	1.9	1.9	..
Sudan	..	0.3	..	..	..	..	..	..	..	..	..	..	..	..	2.7	..	..	..	..	..	..
Suriname	5.9	5.6	4.9	..	4.0	..	..	3.5	3.2	2.5	..	2.0	..	..	2.4	2.4	2.4	2.4	2.0	..	..
Swaziland	..	..	..	..	..	..	..	2.1	2.4	2.5	..	2.8	2.8	..	..	..	..	..	..	..	..
Sweden	8.8	8.7	7.8	7.9	7.6	7.2	7.3	7.9	7.6	6.6	6.6	6.3	5.9	5.9	0.9	1.0	1.1	1.3	1.3	1.3	1.5
Switzerland	8.3	8.9	9.3	9.4	9.4	9.8	..	5.7	6.1	6.5	6.7	6.8	7.0	..	2.6	2.8	2.8	2.6	2.7	2.7	..
Syrian Arab Republic	..	..	..	..	..	..	..	..	..	..	..	..	..	..	..	..	..	..	..	..	..
Taiwan, China	4.2	4.5	4.8	4.9	..	..	..	2.1	2.4	2.6	2.6	..	..	..	2.0	2.2	2.3	2.3	..	..	..
Tajikistan	..	..	..	..	..	..	..	4.3	4.1	4.7	4.9	5.8	..	..	..	..	..	..	..	..	..
Tanzania	..	..	..	..	..	..	..	..	..	..	..	2.2	2.5	..	..	..	..	..	..	..	..
Thailand	..	..	5.3	..	..	..	..	0.9	1.1	1.4	..	..	..	..	..	..	..	..	3.9	..	..
Togo	..	3.4	..	..	..	..	..	1.3	1.2	1.0	0.7	1.7	1.6	..	..	2.2	..	..	..	..	..
Tonga	..	..	..	..	..	..	..	3.7	4.2	4.0	..	..	..	..	..	..	..	..	..	..	..
Trinidad and Tobago	3.8	3.9	3.9	3.8	3.4	..	..	2.3	2.4	2.5	2.4	2.1	2.1	..	1.5	1.5	1.4	1.4	1.3	1.3	..
Tunisia	5.6	..	..	5.9	..	..	..	3.0	..	..	3.0	..	..	..	2.5	..	..	2.8	..	..	..
Turkey	..	..	3.9	..	4.2	..	..	..	..	2.5	..	2.7	..	..	..	..	1.3	..	1.5	..	..
Turkmenistan	..	..	..	..	..	..	..	3.9	3.7	2.0	1.8	1.2	..	..	..	..	..	..	..	..	..
Turks and Caicos Islands	5.5	5.7	5.8	4.7	4.8	..	..	3.3	3.6	3.7	2.5	2.6	2.8	..	2.1	2.1	2.1	2.3	2.2	..	..
Uganda	..	..	..	..	3.9	..	..	..	..	..	2.3	1.8	1.5	..	1.8	..	..	..	2.1	..	..
Ukraine	..	..	..	..	..	..	..	3.0	3.3	3.5	4.1	5.4	4.9	..	..	..	..	..	..	..	..
United Arab Emirates	..	..	..	..	2.5	..	..	..	..	..	..	2.0	..	..	..	..	..	..	0.5	..	..
United Kingdom	6.0	6.5	6.9	6.9	6.9	6.9	6.9	5.1	5.4	5.9	5.8	5.8	5.9	5.8	1.0	1.1	1.1	1.1	1.1	1.1	1.1
United States	12.6	13.3	13.8	14.1	14.0	14.1	14.0	5.1	5.6	5.9	6.1	6.3	6.5	6.6	7.4	7.7	7.9	8.0	7.7	7.6	7.4
Uruguay	7.4	6.3	6.4	6.4	13.4	..	..	3.0	1.4	1.6	1.6	7.0	..	..	4.4	5.0	4.9	4.8	6.5	..	..
Uzbekistan	..	..	..	..	..	..	..	4.6	4.5	4.8	4.1	3.5	..	..	..	..	..	..	..	..	..
Vanuatu	..	..	..	..	..	..	..	2.6	3.0	3.1	3.3	..	..	..	..	..	..	..	..	..	..
Venezuela	6.9	7.4	7.4	7.4	7.5	..	..	2.0	2.9	2.8	2.8	3.0	1.0	..	4.8	4.6	4.6	4.6	4.5	..	..
Vietnam	2.8	..	..	5.2	..	..	..	0.9	..	..	1.1	..	..	..	2.0	..	..	4.1	..	..	..
Virgin Islands (UK)	4.3	4.6	4.2	4.1	4.5	..	..	1.9	2.2	1.7	1.7	2.0	1.9	..	2.4	2.4	2.5	2.5	2.5	..	..
Virgin Islands (US)	..	..	..	..	..	..	..	..	..	..	..	..	..	..	..	..	..	..	..	..	..
West Bank and Gaza	..	10.4	..	..	..	7.0	..	..	6.1	..	..	..	3.2	..	..	4.2	..	..	..	3.8	..
Yemen, Rep.	2.5	..	..	..	2.5	..	..	1.2	..	..	..	1.1	1.1	..	1.4	..	..	..	1.4	..	..
Yugoslavia, Fed. Rep.	..	..	..	..	..	..	..	..	..	..	..	..	..	..	..	..	..	..	..	..	..
Zambia	3.3	..	..	..	..	..	..	2.6	1.5	1.4	1.7	2.1	3.0	..	0.7	..	..	..	..	..	..
Zimbabwe	..	6.2	..	..	..	..	..	..	2.2	2.0	..	2.0	..	..	..	4.0	..	..	..	..	..

Table 3. Health Financing by Expenditure Categories

	Percent of total health expenditure											
	Hospital				Pharmaceutical				Public			
	Total		Public		Total		Public		Capital investment		Personnel	
Economy	Year	Percent	Year	Percent	Year	Percent	Year	Percent	Year	Percent	Year	Percent
Afghanistan		..		..		..		..		..		..
Albania		..		..		..		..		..		..
Algeria		..		..	1993	33	1993	12	1993	3		..
Angola		..		..		..		..		..		..
Anguilla		..		..		..		..		..		..
Antigua and Barbuda		..		..		..		..		..		..
Argentina		..		..		..		..				..
Armenia		..		..		..	1995	9		..	1995	9
Aruba		..		..		..		..		..		..
Australia	1993	43		..	1993	11	1992	5	1993	3		..
Austria	1994	33		..	1994	10	1993	7	1994	5		..
Azerbaijan		..		..		..	1995	2	1995	1	1995	6
Bahamas, The		..		..		..		..		..		..
Bahrain		..		..		..		..		..		..
Bangladesh	1995	14	1995	14				..	1995	27		..
Barbados		..		..		..		..		..		..
Belarus		..		..		..	1995	14	1995	14	1995	27
Belgium	1994	36		..	1995	19	1993	8		..		..
Belize		..		..		..		..	1990	13		..
Benin		..		..		..		..		..		..
Bermuda		..		..		..		..		..		..
Bhutan		..		..		..		..	1991	9		..
Bolivia		..		..		..		..		..		..
Bosnia and Herzegovina		..		..		..		..		..		..
Botswana		..	1991	21		..		..	1991	14		..
Brazil		..		..		..		..		..		..
Brunei		..		..		..		..		..		..
Bulgaria		..		..		..	1992	15	1992	4	1992	35
Burkina Faso		..		..		..		..	1992	10	1992	12
Burundi		..		..		..		..		..		..
Cambodia		..		..		..		..		..		..
Cameroon		..		..	1995	14	1993	4	1994	5	1994	40
Canada	1994	47		..	1995	14	1993	4	1994	2		..
Cape Verde		..		..		..		..		..		..
Cayman Islands		..		..		..		..		..		..
Central African Republic		..		..		..		..		..		..
Chad		..		..		..		..		..		..
Channel Islands		..		..		..		..		..		..
Chile		..		..		..		..	1990	4		..
China	1993	31	1993	17	1993	53	1993	24	1993	1		..
Colombia		..		..		..		..		..		..
Comoros		..		..		..		..		..	1993	61
Congo, Dem. Rep.		..		..		..		..				..
Congo, Rep.		..		..		..		..	1992	1		..
Costa Rica		..		..		..		..	1990	0		..
Côte d'Ivoire		..		..		..		..		..		..
Croatia		..	1994	36		..	1994	21	1994	1	1994	21
Cuba		..		..		..		..		..		..
Cyprus		..		..		..		..		..		..
Czech Republic		..		..		..	1994	10	1995	3	1994	23
Denmark	1994	61		..	1994	11	1993	6	1994	4		..
Djibouti		..		..		..		..		..		..
Dominica		..		..		..		..		..		..
Dominican Republic		..		..		..		..	1990	23		..
Ecuador		..		..		..		..	1990	6		..
Egypt, Arab Rep.		..		..	1990	43		..		..	1990	9
El Salvador		..		..		..		..		..		..
Equatorial Guinea		..		..		..		..		..		..
Eritrea	1994	40	1994	39		..		..		..		..
Estonia		..		..		..		..		..		..
Ethiopia		..		..		..		..		..		..
Fiji		..		..	1992	18	1992	6		..		..
Finland	1994	41		..	1994	13	1993	6	1994	3		..
France	1994	45		..	1995	17	1993	10	1994	3		..
French Guiana		..		..		..		..		..		..
French Polynesia		..		..		..		..		..		..
Gabon		..		..		..		..		..		..
Gambia, The		..		..		..		..		..		..
Georgia		..		..		..		..		..		..
Germany	1993	31		..	1993	19	1992	13	1993	4		..
Ghana		..		..		..		..		..		..
Greece	1992	59		..	1992	24	1991	7	1992	3		..
Grenada		..		..		..		..		..		..
Guadeloupe		..		..		..		..		..		..
Guam		..		..		..		..		..		..

Table 3. Health Financing by Expenditure Categories (*continued*)

	Percent of total health expenditure											
	Hospital				Pharmaceutical				Public			
	Total		Public		Total		Public		Capital investment		Personnel	
Economy	Year	Percent	Year	Percent	Year	Percent	Year	Percent	Year	Percent	Year	Percent
Guatemala		..		..		..		..		..		..
Guinea		..		..		..		..		..		..
Guinea-Bissau		..		..		..		..		..		..
Guyana		..		..		..		..		..		..
Haiti		..		..		..		..		..		..
Honduras		..		..		..		..	1990	35		..
Hong Kong, China		..		..		..		..	1994	5		
Hungary		..	1994	34		..	1994	28	1994	6	1994	30
Iceland	1995	68		..	1995	16	1994	11	1995	2		..
India		..	1992	6		..		..	1992	2	1992	12
Indonesia		..	1994	4		..	1994	2	1994	26	1994	15
Iran, Islamic Rep.		..		..		..		..		..		..
Iraq		..		..		..		..		..		..
Ireland		..		..	1994	12	1992	9	1993	2		..
Israel		..		..		..		..		..		..
Italy	1995	48		..	1995	18	1994	7	1995	1		..
Jamaica		..		..		..		..	1990	3		
Japan	1993	32		..		..		..	1993	5		
Jordan	1994	36		..	1994	27		..	1994	5		
Kazakhstan		..		..		..		..		..		..
Kenya		..		..		..		..	1992	11		..
Kiribati		..		..		..		..		..		..
Korea, Dem. Rep.		..		..		..		..		..		..
Korea, Rep.		..		..	1992	24		..		..		..
Kuwait		..		..		..		..		..		..
Kyrgyz Republic		..		..		..		..		..		..
Lao PDR		..		..		..	1995	3	1995	4	1995	18
Latvia		..		..		..		..		..		..
Lebanon		..		..		..	1992	1		..	1992	2
Lesotho		..		..		..		..		..		..
Liberia		..		..		..		..		..		..
Libya		..		..		..		..		..		..
Lithuania		..		..		..		..		..		..
Luxembourg	1994	32		..	1991	16	1991	15				..
Macao		..		..		..		..		..		..
Macedonia, FYR		..		..		..	1995	13	1995	2	1995	48
Madagascar		..		..		..		..		..		..
Malawi		..		..		..		..		..		..
Malaysia		..		..		..		..		..		..
Maldives		..		..		..		..		..		..
Mali		..		..		..		..	1991	24		..
Malta		..		..		..		..		..		..
Marshall Islands		..		..		..		..		..		..
Martinique		..		..		..		..		..		..
Mauritania		..		..		..		..	1991	5	1991	12
Mauritius		..		..		..		..		..		..
Mayotte		..		..		..		..		..		..
Mexico		..		..		..		..		..		..
Micronesia, Fed. Sts.		..		..		..		..		..		..
Moldova		..		..		..		..		..		..
Mongolia		..		..		..	1992	1	1992	8	1992	28
Montserrat		..		..		..		..		..		..
Morocco		..	1993	24	1993	65	1993	4	1993	8	1993	19
Mozambique		..		..		..		..		..		..
Myanmar		..		..		..		..		..		..
Namibia		..	1993	21		..	1993	0		..	1993	30
Nepal		..		..		..		..	1995	1		..
Netherlands	1994	52		..	1995	11	1993	10		..		..
Netherlands Antilles		..		..		..		..		..		..
New Caledonia		..		..		..		..		..		..
New Zealand	1993	59		..	1993	17	1992	11	1993	4		..
Nicaragua		..		..		..		..		..		..
Niger		..		..		..		..		..		..
Nigeria		..		..		..		..	1994	8	1994	17
Norway	1991	67		..	1991	11	1990	5	1993	5		..
Oman		..		..		..		..		..		..
Pakistan		..	1991	10		..		..	1991	8		..
Panama		..		..		..		..		..		..
Papua New Guinea		..		..		..		..		..		..
Paraguay		..		..		..		..		..		..
Peru		..		..		..		..		..		..
Philippines		..		..		..		..		..		..
Poland		..	1992	40		..	1992	14	1992	6	1992	42
Portugal		..		..		..	1993	2		..	1994	25
Puerto Rico		..		..		..		..		..		..

Table 3. Health Financing by Expenditure Categories (*continued*)

	Hospital				Pharmaceutical				Public			
	Total		Public		Total		Public		Capital investment		Personnel	
Economy	Year	Percent	Year	Percent	Year	Percent	Year	Percent	Year	Percent	Year	Percent
Qatar		..		..		..		..		..		..
Reunion		..		..		..		..		..		..
Romania		..		..		..		..		..		..
Russian Federation		..	1994	38		..	1994	11	1991	15	1991	46
Rwanda		..		..		..		..		..		
Samoa		..		..		..		..		..		..
São Tomé and Principe		..		..		..		..		..		..
Saudi Arabia		..		..		..		..		..		..
Senegal		..		..		..		..		..		..
Seychelles		..		..		..		..		..		..
Sierra Leone		..		..		..		..		..		..
Singapore		..		..		..		..		..		..
Slovak Republic		..		..		..		..		..		..
Slovenia		..		..		..		..		..		..
Solomon Islands		..		..		..		..	1991	7		..
Somalia		..		..		..		..		..		..
South Africa		..	1993	28		..		..		..		..
Spain	1993	49		..	1992	18	1992	15	1992	3		..
Sri Lanka		..		..		..		..	1993	16		..
St. Kitts and Nevis		..		..		..		..		..		..
St. Lucia		..		..		..		..		..		..
St. Vincent and the Grenadines		..		..		..		..		..		..
Sudan		..		..		..		..		..		..
Suriname		..		..		..		..		..		..
Swaziland		..		..		..		..		..		..
Sweden		..		..	1994	13	1994	11	1994	3		
Switzerland	1992	51		..	1992	7	1991	5	1992	3		..
Syrian Arab Republic		..		..		..		..		..		..
Taiwan, China		..		..		..		..	1993	4		..
Tajikistan		..		..		..		..		..		..
Tanzania		..		..		..		..		..		..
Thailand		..		..		..		..		..		..
Togo		..		..		..		..		..	1991	24
Tonga		..		..		..	1992	7	1992	8	1992	46
Trinidad and Tobago		..		..		..		..		..		..
Tunisia		..		..		..		..		..		..
Turkey	1994	26		..	1994	27		..		..		..
Turkmenistan		..		..		..		..		..		..
Turks and Caicos Islands		..		..		..		..		..		..
Uganda		..	1994	21		..		..	1994	12		
Ukraine		..		..		..		..		..		..
United Arab Emirates		..		..		..		..	1994	14	1994	43
United Kingdom	1993	43		..	1995	16	1993	10	1994	4		..
United States	1994	43		..	1995	9	1993	1	1993	0		..
Uruguay		..		..		..		..		..		..
Uzbekistan		..		..		..		..		..		..
Vanuatu		..		..		..		..		..		..
Venezuela		..		..		..		..		..		..
Vietnam	1993	55	1993	18	1993	99	1993	39	1993	1	1990	9
Virgin Islands (UK)		..		..		..		..		..		..
Virgin Islands (US)		..		..		..		..		..		..
West Bank and Gaza	1995	32	1991	35	1995	36	1995	7				..
Yemen, Rep.		..		..	1994	72	1994	14	1994	4	1990	27
Yugoslavia, Fed. Rep.		..		..		..		..		..		..
Zambia		..		..		..		..	1990	4	1990	30
Zimbabwe		..		..		..		..	1991	0	1991	15

27

Table 4. Sources of Health Financing

Economy	Year	Percent total health expenditure			
		Total public	Social health insurance	Government budget[a]	External grants and borrowings
Afghanistan		..	..	..	..
Albania		..	..	..	..
Algeria	1993	73	37	36	..
Angola		..	..	..	..
Anguilla	1994	47	..	47	..
Antigua and Barbuda	1994	61	..	61	..
Argentina	1994	40	25	15	..
Armenia	1995	40	..	25	15
Aruba		..	..	..	..
Australia	1994	68	8	61	..
Austria	1994	76	58	18	..
Azerbaijan	1995	18	..	18	..
Bahamas, The	1994	59	..	59	..
Bahrain		..	..	..	..
Bangladesh	1995	48	..	31	17
Barbados	1994	65	..	65	..
Belarus	1995	83	..	83	..
Belgium	1995	88	..	88	..
Belize	1994	75	..	75	..
Benin		..	..	..	..
Bermuda	1994	15	..	15	..
Bhutan	1991	46	..	46	..
Bolivia	1994	53	20	33	..
Bosnia and Herzegovina		..	..	..	..
Botswana	1991	55	..	55	..
Brazil	1994	36	..	36	..
Brunei		..	..	..	..
Bulgaria	1992	80	..	80	..
Burkina Faso	1992	42	..	30	12
Burundi		..	..	..	..
Cambodia	1994	10	..	10	..
Cameroon	1994	72	..	56	15
Canada	1994	72	12	60	..
Cape Verde		..	..	..	..
Cayman Islands	1994	58	..	58	..
Central African Republic		..	..	..	..
Chad		97	..	..	77
Channel Islands		..	..	..	..
Chile	1994	39	28	11	..
China	1993	54	31	23	..
Colombia	1994	40	19	20	1
Comoros	1993	79	..	79	..
Cong, Dem. Rep.		..	..	..	..
Congo, Rep.	1992	50	..	43	7
Costa Rica	1994	74	60	14	..
Côte d'Ivoire	1995	40	3	29	8
Croatia	1994	84	65	18	..
Cuba		..	..	..	..
Cyprus		..	..	..	..
Czech Republic	1995	80	68	13	..
Denmark	1994	83	..	83	..
Djibouti		..	..	..	..
Dominica		..	..	..	..
Dominican Republic	1994	38	10	28	..
Ecuador	1994	39	18	21	..
Egypt, Arab Rep.	1990	41	9	31	2
El Salvador	1994	24	12	12	..
Equatorial Guinea	1990	81	..	37	44
Eritrea	1994	55	..	55	..
Estonia		..	..	..	..
Ethiopia		61	1	43	17
Fiji	1992	68	..	61	8
Finland	1994	75	10	65	..
France	1995	81	..	81	..
French Guiana		..	..	..	..
French Polynesia		..	..	..	..
Gabon		..	..	..	..
Gambia, The		..	..	..	..
Georgia		..	..	..	..
Germany	1995	78	..	78	..
Ghana	1995	93	..	54	39
Greece	1993	76	..	76	..
Grenada		..	..	..	..
Guadeloupe		..	..	..	..
Guam		..	..	..	..

Table 4. Sources of Health Financing (*continued*)

| Economy | Year | Percent total health expenditure | | | |
		Total public	Social health insurance	Government budget[a]	External grants and borrowings
Guatemala	1994	35	..	35	..
Guinea		..	..	..	..
Guinea-Bissau		..	..	..	..
Guyana		..	..	..	..
Haiti	1994	36	..	36	..
Honduras	1994	50	18	32	..
Hong Kong, China	1994	44	..	44	..
Hungary	1994	93	70	23	..
Iceland	1995	84	..	84	..
India	1992	22	2	18	3
Indonesia	1994	37	..	31	5
Iran, Islamic Rep.	1990	58	12	46	..
Iraq		..	..	..	..
Ireland	1994	81	7	74	..
Israel	1990	50	..	50	..
Italy	1995	70	..	70	..
Jamaica	1994	57	..	53	4
Japan	1994	77	..	77	..
Jordan	1994	47	..	47	..
Kazakhstan		..	..	..	..
Kenya	1992	62	9	52	..
Kiribati		..	..	..	..
Korea, Dem. Rep.		..	..	..	..
Korea, Rep.	1992	33	23	10	..
Kuwait		..	..	..	..
Kyrgyz Republic		..	..	..	..
Lao PDR	1995	48	..	32	17
Latvia		..	..	..	..
Lebanon	1992	39	16	15	8
Lesotho		..	..	..	..
Liberia		..	..	..	..
Libya		..	..	..	..
Lithuania		..	..	..	..
Luxembourg	1993	93	..	93	..
Macao		..	..	..	..
Macedonia, FYR	1995	89	72	17	..
Madagascar		..	..	..	..
Malawi		..	..	..	..
Malaysia	1993	60	..	60	..
Maldives		..	..	..	..
Mali	1991	46	..	22	24
Malta		..	..	..	..
Marshall Islands		..	..	..	..
Martinique		..	..	..	..
Mauritania	1991	21	..	17	4
Mauritius	1991	62	..	62	..
Mayotte		..	..	..	..
Mexico	1994	52	23	29	..
Micronesia, Fed. Sts.		..	..	..	..
Moldova		..	..	..	..
Mongolia	1992	92	2	90	..
Montserrat	1994	56	..	56	..
Morocco	1993	48	15	30	2
Mozambique		..	..	..	..
Myanmar		..	..	..	..
Namibia	1993	52	..	52	..
Nepal	1995	24	..	11	14
Netherlands	1995	77	..	77	..
Netherlands Antilles	1994	53	..	53	..
New Caledonia		..	..	..	..
New Zealand	1994	77	5	72	..
Nicaragua	1994	55	..	55	..
Niger		..	..	..	..
Nigeria	1994	25	..	25	..
Norway	1994	83	..	83	..
Oman		..	..	..	..
Pakistan	1991	22	..	22	..
Panama	1994	73	46	27	..
Papua New Guinea		..	..	..	..
Paraguay	1994	23	..	23	..
Peru	1994	53	33	20	..
Philippines	1991	56	12	44	..
Poland	1992	83	..	83	..
Portugal	1995	60	..	60	..
Puerto Rico		..	..	..	..

Table 4. Sources of Health Financing (*continued*)

Economy	Year	Total public	Percent total health expenditure Social health insurance	Government budget[a]	External grants and borrowings
Qatar		..	..	..	..
Reunion		..	..	..	..
Romania		..	..	..	..
Russian Federation	1991	93	18	75	..
Rwanda		..	..	..	..
Samoa		..	..	..	..
São Tomé and Principe		..	..	..	..
Saudi Arabia		..	..	..	..
Senegal		..	..	..	..
Seychelles		..	..	..	..
Sierra Leone	1991	43	..	9	33
Singapore	1994	33	7	25	..
Slovak Republic		..	..	..	..
Slovenia		..	..	..	..
Solomon Islands	1991	86	..	60	26
Somalia		..	..	..	..
South Africa	1993	45	..	45	0
Spain	1995	79	21	57	..
Sri Lanka	1993	76	..	76	..
St. Kitts and Nevis	1994	58	..	58	..
St. Lucia		..	..	..	..
St. Vincent and the Grenadines	1994	67	..	67	..
Sudan		..	..	..	..
Suriname	1994	51	13	38	..
Swaziland		..	..	..	..
Sweden	1994	83	..	83	..
Switzerland	1994	70	42	28	..
Syrian Arab Republic		..	..	..	..
Taiwan, China	1993	54	39	15	..
Tajikistan		..	..	..	..
Tanzania		..	..	..	..
Thailand	1992	26	..	26	..
Togo	1991	35	..	34	2
Tonga	1992	73	..	45	27
Trinidad and Tobago	1994	67	..	67	..
Tunisia	1993	52	14	37	..
Turkey	1994	65	20	45	..
Turkmenistan		..	..	..	..
Turks and Caicos Islands		..	..	..	..
Uganda	1994	45	..	21	24
Ukraine		..	..	..	..
United Arab Emirates	1994	81	..	81	..
United Kingdom	1994	84	10	74	..
United States	1995	45	14	31	..
Uruguay	1994	24	..	24	..
Uzbekistan		..	..	..	..
Vanuatu					
Venezuela	1994	33	7	25	..
Vietnam	1993	22	2	20	..
Virgin Islands (UK)	1994	53	..	53	..
Virgin Islands (US)		..	..	..	..
West Bank and Gaza	1995	46	9	17	20
Yemen, Rep.	1994	43	..	43	..
Yugoslavia, Fed. Rep.		..	..	..	..
Zambia	1990	78	..	71	7
Zimbabwe	1991	35	..	35	..

a. May include external grants and borrowings.

Table 5. Health Services Indicators, 1990–95

Economy	Year	Inpatient beds per 1,000 population			Year	Physicians per 1,000 population		
		Total	Year	Public		Total	Year	Public
Afghanistan	1990	0.2		..	1993	0.14		..
Albania	1995	3.2		..	1995	1.40		..
Algeria	1994	2.1	1994	2.1	1993	0.82		..
Angola	1990	1.3	1990	1.2	1990	0.04		..
Anguilla		..		..	1990–95	1.10		..
Antigua and Barbuda	1993	6.1		..	1993	3.03		..
Argentina	1990	4.6		..	1990	2.68		..
Armenia	1992	8.4		..	1995	3.05		..
Aruba		..		..	1990–95	1.10		..
Australia	1993	8.9	1991	6.0	1991	2.20		..
Austria	1995	9.3		..	1994	2.60		..
Azerbaijan	1994	10.0	1994	10.1	1994	3.86	1994	3.90
Bahamas, The	1993	3.9		..	1993	1.45		..
Bahrain		..		..	1991	1.31		..
Bangladesh	1994	0.3	1995	0.2	1995	0.20		..
Barbados	1990	8.4		..	1990	1.14		..
Belarus	1995	11.6		..	1995	4.09		..
Belgium	1994	7.6	1992	3.0	1994	3.70		..
Belize	1993	2.8		..	1993	0.53		..
Benin	1994	0.2		..	1994	0.06		..
Bermuda		..		..	1990–95	1.20		..
Bhutan	1994	1.6		..	1994	0.16		..
Bolivia	1991	1.4		..	1993	0.43		..
Bosnia and Herzegovina	1995	1.8		..	1995	0.52		..
Botswana	1990	1.6		..	1993	0.19	1990	1.57
Brazil	1995	3.0		..	1995	1.42		..
Brunei		..		..	1991	..		..
Bulgaria	1995	10.6	1994	10.2	1995	3.46		..
Burkina Faso	1990	0.3		..		..		..
Burundi	1991	0.7		..	1991	0.06		..
Cambodia	1990	2.1	1994	0.9	1994	0.10		..
Cameroon	1990	2.6		..	1992	0.08	1990	0.08
Canada	1995	5.1	1992	5.8	1994	2.20		..
Cape Verde	1992	1.6	1990	1.2	1992	0.23	1990	0.34
Cayman Islands	1990	3.0		..	1990	1.70		..
Central African Republic	1990	0.9		..	1990	0.04	1990	0.04
Chad	1991	0.7		..		..	1990	0.34
Channel Islands		..		..		..		..
Chile	1990	3.1		..	1991	1.06		..
China	1994	2.4		..	1994	1.57		..
Colombia	1990	1.4		..	1993	0.90		..
Comoros	1990	2.8		..	1990	0.11		..
Congo, Dem. Rep.	1990	1.4		..	1990	0.07		..
Congo, Rep.	1990	3.3		..	1990	0.27		..
Costa Rica	1990	2.5		..	1993	0.88		..
Côte d'Ivoire	1990	0.8		..	1990	0.09	1990	0.09
Croatia	1994	5.9	1994	5.9	1994	2.01	1994	2.01
Cuba	1990	5.4		..	1990	3.64		..
Cyprus		..		..	1990	1.76		..
Czech Republic	1995	9.2	1994	9.8	1995	2.99		..
Denmark	1994	5.0		..	1994	2.90		..
Djibouti	1990	2.6		..	1990	0.17	1990	0.19
Dominica	1993	2.6		..	1991	0.53		..
Dominican Republic	1993	2.0		..	1993	1.05		..
Ecuador	1990	1.6		..		..		..
Egypt, Arab Rep.	1993	1.9	1992	1.8	1994	1.84	1994	0.92
El Salvador	1990	1.5		..	1993	0.66		..
Equatorial Guinea		..		..	1990	0.28		..
Eritrea		..		..		..		..
Estonia	1994	8.0		..	1995	3.08	1993	3.31
Ethiopia	1990	0.2	1990	0.2	1994	0.03	1990	0.03
Fiji		..		..	1992	0.48	1992	0.34
Finland	1994	10.1	1994	9.6	1994	2.70		..
France	1994	9.0	1994	5.8	1994	2.80		..
French Guiana		..		..	1990–95	1.30		..
French Polynesia		..		..		..		..
Gabon	1990	3.3		..	1993	0.50		..
Gambia, The	1990	0.6		..		..	1990	0.07
Georgia	1994	8.2		..	1993	4.14		..
Germany	1993	9.7	1992	5.2	1994	3.30		..
Ghana	1990	1.5	1990	1.2		..	1991	0.05
Greece	1994	5.0	1992	3.5	1994	4.00		..
Grenada	1993	8.1		..	1993	0.57		..
Guadeloupe		..		..	1990–95	1.40		..
Guam		..		..		..		..

Table 5. Health Services Indicators, 1990–95 (continued)

Economy	Year	Inpatient beds per 1,000 population Total	Year	Public	Year	Physicians per 1,000 population Total	Year	Public
Guatemala	1990	1.1		..	1993	0.25		..
Guinea	1990	0.6		..	1994	0.15		..
Guinea-Bissau	1990	1.5		..		..		..
Guyana	1993	2.8		..	1993	0.11		..
Haiti	1993	0.8		..	1993	0.09		..
Honduras	1990	1.0		..	1991	0.41		..
Hong Kong, China	1990	4.3	1994	4.1	1995	1.31	1994	0.53
Hungary	1994	9.9	1994	9.9	1994	3.37	1994	3.43
Iceland	1992	15.9		..	1994	3.00		..
India	1991	0.8		..	1993	0.41		..
Indonesia	1994	0.7	1994	0.4	1994	0.17		..
Iran, Islamic Republic	1990	1.4		..	1993	0.32		..
Iraq	1990	1.7		..	1993	0.60		..
Ireland	1994	5.0		..	1994	2.00		..
Israel	1995	3.2	1988–92	..		..		..
Italy	1993	6.7	1991	5.4	1992	1.70		..
Jamaica	1993	2.1		..	1993	0.47		..
Japan	1994	16.2	1994	5.1	1994	1.80		..
Jordan	1994	1.6		..	1994	1.64		..
Kazakhstan	1995	11.6	1994	12.1	1995	3.62	1994	3.60
Kenya	1990	1.7	1990	1.4	1990	0.05	1990	0.14
Kiribati	1990	4.3		..	1992	0.19		..
Korea, Dem. Rep.		..		..		..		..
Korea, Rep.	1994	4.1		..	1994	1.22		..
Kuwait		..		..	1990	0.04		..
Kyrgyz Republic	1993	10.9	1994	9.6	1995	3.18	1994	3.10
Lao PDR	1990	2.5	1993	1.1	1990	0.22		..
Latvia	1993	12.1		..	1995	2.94		..
Lebanon	1992	4.0	1992	0.2	1991	1.33		..
Lesotho		..	1994	1.4	1990	0.04	1994	0.06
Liberia		..		..		..		..
Libya	1990	4.1		..	1990	1.04		..
Lithuania	1992	11.9	1994	11.1	1995	3.97		..
Luxembourg	1993	11.5		..	1993	2.20		..
Macao		..		..		..		..
Macedonia, FYR	1995	5.0		..	1995	2.13		..
Madagascar	1990	0.9	1990	0.9	1990	0.12	1990	0.12
Malawi	1990	1.6		..	1990	0.02	1990	0.02
Malaysia	1994	2.0	1994	1.7	1994	0.45	1993	0.20
Maldives	1990	0.8		..	1990	0.07		..
Mali		..		..	1990	0.05	1990	0.05
Malta	1995	5.4		..	1993	2.50		..
Marshall Islands	1990	2.3		..		..	1992	0.38
Martinique		..		..	1990–95	1.70		..
Mauritania	1990	0.7		..	1993	0.06	1990	0.06
Mauritius	1994	3.1	1994	2.9	1995	0.86	1995	0.86
Mayotte		..		..		..		..
Mexico	1994	1.2	1994	0.6	1994	1.30	1992	1.15
Micronesia, Fed. Sts.		..		..		..		..
Moldova	1995	12.2		..	1995	3.51		..
Mongolia	1991	11.5	1994	9.5	1991	2.70	1994	2.47
Montserrat		..		..	1990–95	0.50		..
Morocco	1994	1.1		..	1994	0.36		..
Mozambique	1990	0.9		..		..	1991	0.03
Myanmar	1990	0.6		..	1990	0.08		..
Namibia	1990	5.0	1995	0.5	1991	0.23	1990	0.22
Nepal	1994	0.2		..	1993	0.07		..
Netherlands	1994	11.3		..	1990	2.50		..
Netherlands Antilles		..		..	1990–95	1.40		..
New Caledonia		..		..		..		..
New Zealand	1992	7.3		..	1994	2.10		..
Nicaragua	1990	1.8		..	1990	0.66		..
Niger		..	1990	0.5	1990	0.02	1990	0.02
Nigeria	1990	1.7	1990	1.1	1993	0.19	1990	0.20
Norway		..		..	1993	3.30		..
Oman	1990	2.1		..	1990	0.61		..
Pakistan	1993	0.7	1990	0.5	1993	0.52		..
Panama	1990	2.5		..	1993	1.78		..
Papua New Guinea	1990	4.0		..	1990	0.07	1990	0.07
Paraguay	1994	0.6		..	1994	0.28		..
Peru	1994	1.4	1994	1.1	1992	1.03		..
Philippines	1993	1.1	1993	0.5	1990	0.12	1993	0.11
Poland	1993	6.4	1994	5.4	1994	2.28	1994	2.20
Portugal	1994	4.3	1994	3.4	1994	2.90	1994	2.90
Puerto Rico		..		..	1990–95	1.80		..

Table 5. Health Services Indicators, 1990–95 (*continued*)

Economy	Year	Inpatient beds per 1,000 population Total	Year	Public	Year	Physicians per 1,000 population Total	Year	Public
Qatar		..		..	1990	1.50		..
Reunion		..				..		..
Romania	1994	7.7	1994	7.7	1994	1.76	1994	1.76
Russian Federation	1995	11.7		..	1995	3.80		..
Rwanda	1990	1.7		..	1993.0	0.04	1990	0.24
Samoa		..		..		..		..
São Tomé and Principe	1991	4.8		..	1990	0.54		..
Saudi Arabia	1990	2.5		..	1990	1.43		
Senegal	1990	0.7		..	1990	0.05	1995	0.07
Seychelles		..	1990	6.2	1991	5.97	1990	0.69
Sierra Leone		..		..		..		..
Singapore	1994	3.6	1994	2.8	1994	1.41	1994	0.70
Slovak Republic	1995	7.6	1994	7.1	1995	3.03	1994	3.00
Slovenia	1995	5.7	1993	5.0	1993	2.05	1993	2.03
Solomon Islands	1992	2.8	1992	2.2	1992	0.16	1992	0.15
Somalia	1990	0.7		..		..		
South Africa		..	1993	4.0		..	1993	0.61
Spain	1991	4.2	1991	3.5	1993	4.10		..
Sri Lanka	1990	2.7	1994	2.8	1993	0.15	1994	0.22
St. Kitts and Nevis	1990	9.2		..	1990	0.90		..
St. Lucia	1993	4.3		..	1993	0.53		..
St. Vincent and the Grenadines	1993	5.0		..	1991	0.51		..
Sudan	1990	1.1		..		..		..
Suriname	1990	5.7		..	1993	0.79		..
Swaziland		..		..	1990	0.10		..
Sweden	1995	6.3	1994	5.2	1995	3.10		..
Switzerland	1991	20.8		..	1994	3.10		..
Syrian Arab Republic	1990	1.1		..	1990	0.83		..
Taiwan, China	1994	4.9		..	1994	1.29		..
Tajikistan	1994	8.8	1994	8.8	1994	2.09	1994	2.10
Tanzania	1992	0.9	1992	0.5		..	1990	0.04
Thailand	1992	1.7	1992	1.5	1992	0.24	1992	0.19
Togo	1990	1.5	1990	1.5	1991	0.09	1991	0.09
Tonga		..	1992	3.3	1991	0.53		..
Trinidad and Tobago	1993	3.2		..	1993	0.66		
Tunisia	1994	1.8	1991	1.9	1993	0.65	1993	0.32
Turkey	1994	2.5	1993	2.4	1994	1.10		..
Turkmenistan	1994	11.5		..	1994	3.24	1994	3.53
Turks and Caicos Islands		..		..	1990–95	0.50		..
Uganda	1991	0.9		..		..	1991	0.04
Ukraine	1995	11.8		..	1995	4.38		..
United Arab Emirates	1992	3.1	1992	0.3	1992	0.84		..
United Kingdom	1993	5.1	1993	4.9	1993	1.50		..
United States	1992	4.4	1990	0.9	1993	2.50		..
Uruguay	1990	4.5		..	1992	3.23		..
Uzbekistan	1995	8.4	1994	8.8	1995	3.26		..
Vanuatu		..		..	1991	0.10	1991	0.10
Venezuela	1992	2.6		..	1990	1.58		..
Vietnam	1990	3.8	1993	2.6	1992	0.44	1990	0.37
Virgin Islands (UK)		..		..	1990–95	1.70		..
Virgin Islands (US)	1990	4.8		..	1990	1.65		..
West Bank and Gaza		..		..		..		..
Yemen, Rep.	1990	0.8		..	1990	0.10		..
Yugoslavia, Fed. Republic	1990	13.6		..	1990	4.32		..
Zambia		..	1990	1.3	1990	0.09	1990	0.09
Zimbabwe	1990	0.5		..	1990	0.14		..
World		3.3		..		1.31		..
Low-income		1.6		..		0.86		..
Excluding China and India		1.4		..		0.33		..
Middle-income		4.1		..		1.59		..
Low- and middle-income		2.4		..		1.10		..
East Asia and Pacific		2.1		..		1.20		..
Europe and Central Asia		9.2		..		3.13		..
Latin America and the Caribbean		2.4		..		1.37		..
Middle East and North Africa		1.7		..		0.89		..
South Asia		0.7		..		0.38		..
Sub-Saharan Africa		1.2		..		0.11		..
High-income		7.6		..		2.35		..

Table 6. Utilization of Health Services, 1990–95

Economy	Outpatient visits per capita per year				Inpatient admissions (% of population)				Average number of days per stay				Bed occupancy rate (% of total)			
	Year	Total	Year	Public	Year	Total	Year	Public	Year	Total	Year	Public	Year	Total	Year	Public
Afghanistan	..	..		..	..	..		..	..	..		..	..	..		..
Albania	..	..		..	..	..		..	..	..		..	..	..		..
Algeria	..	..		..	..	..		..	..	..		..	..	..	1994	44.0
Angola	..	..		..	..	..		..	..	..		..	..	..		..
Anguilla	..	..		..	..	..		..	..	..		..	..	..		..
Antigua and Barbuda	..	..		..	..	..		..	..	..		..	..	..		..
Argentina	..	..		..	..	..		..	..	..		..	..	..		..
Armenia	..	..		..	..	..		..	..	..		..	..	..		..
Aruba	..	..		..	..	..		..	..	..		..	..	..		..
Australia	1993	10.6		..	1995	13.80		..	1994	14.0		..	1992	74.5		..
Austria	1994	6.2		..	1995	24.70		..	1995	10.9	1994	..	1995	79.4		..
Azerbaijan	..	..		..	..	..		..	..	..	1994	17.9	..	..	1993	65.0
Bahamas, The	..	..		..	..	..		..	..	..		..	..	..		..
Bahrain	..	..		..	..	..		..	..	..		..	..	..		..
Bangladesh	..	..		..	..	..		..	..	..	1995	8.9	1995	79.0		..
Barbados	..	..		..	..	..		..	..	..		..	..	..		..
Belarus	..	..		..	..	..		..	..	..		..	..	..		..
Belgium	1993	8.0		..	1994	19.80		..	1995	11.5		..	1993	83.5		..
Belize	..	..		..	..	..		..	..	..		..	..	..		..
Benin	..	..		..	..	..		..	..	..		..	..	..		..
Bermuda	..	..		..	..	..		..	..	..		..	..	..		..
Bhutan	..	..		..	..	..		..	..	..		..	..	..		..
Bolivia	..	..		..	..	..		..	..	..		..	..	..		..
Bosnia and Herzegovina	..	..		..	..	..		..	..	..		..	..	..		..
Botswana	..	..		..	..	..		..	..	..		..	..	..		..
Brazil	1995	2.3		..	1995	0.10		..	..	..		..	..	..		..
Brunei	..	..		..	..	..		..	..	..		..	..	..		..
Bulgaria	..	..		..	..	..	1994	18.20	..	..	1994	14.1	..	..		..
Burkina Faso	..	..		..	..	..		..	..	..		..	..	..		..
Burundi	..	..		..	..	..		..	..	..		..	..	..		..
Cambodia	..	..		..	..	..		..	..	..		..	..	..		..
Cameroon	..	..		..	..	..		..	..	..		..	..	..		..
Canada	1991	6.9		..	1993	12.50		..	1995	12.2		..	1993	84.2		..
Cape Verde	..	..		..	..	..		..	..	..		..	..	..		..
Cayman Islands	..	..		..	..	..		..	..	..		..	..	..		..
Central African Republic	..	..		..	..	..		..	..	..		..	..	..		..
Chad	..	..		..	..	..		..	..	..		..	..	..		..
Channel Islands	..	..		..	..	..		..	..	..		..	..	..		..
Chile	..	..		..	..	..		..	..	..		..	..	..		..
China	..	..	1994	1.8	1994	4.19		..	1994	15.0		..	1994	69.0		..
Colombia	..	..		..	..	..		..	..	..		..	..	..		..
Comoros	..	..		..	..	..		..	..	..		..	..	..		..
Congo, Dem. Rep.	..	..		..	..	..		..	..	..		..	..	..		..
Congo, Rep.	..	..		..	..	..		..	..	..		..	..	..		..
Costa Rica	..	..		..	..	..		..	..	..		..	..	..		..
Côte d'Ivoire	..	..		..	..	..		..	..	..		..	..	..		..
Croatia	..	..		..	..	..	1994	13.80	..	..		..	..	..		..
Cuba	..	..		..	..	..		..	..	..		..	..	..		..
Cyprus	..	..		..	..	..		..	..	..		..	..	..		..
Czech Republic	..	..		..	1994	20.70	1993	18.70	1995	12.8	1993	11.2	1995	77.6		..
Denmark	1993	4.8		..	1995	25.40		..	1995	7.5		..	1994	83.8		..
Djibouti	..	..		..	..	..		..	..	..		..	..	..		..
Dominica	..	..		..	..	..		..	..	..		..	..	..		..
Dominican Republic	..	..		..	..	..		..	..	..		..	..	..		..
Ecuador	..	..		..	..	..		..	..	..		..	..	..		..
Egypt, Arab Rep.	1994	4.5		..	1994	3.32		..	1994	10.2		..	..	..	1992	49.0
El Salvador	..	..		..	..	..		..	..	..		..	..	..		..
Equatorial Guinea	..	..		..	..	..		..	..	..		..	..	..		..
Eritrea	..	..		..	..	..		..	..	..		..	..	..		..
Estonia	..	..		..	..	..	1993	18.90	..	..	1993	15.4	..	..		..
Ethiopia	..	..		..	..	..		..	..	..		..	..	..		..
Fiji	..	..		..	1990	0.08		..	1990	61.0		..	1990	65.0		..
Finland	1994	4.0		..	1995	22.70		..	1995	11.8		..	1995	87.7		..
France	1993	6.3		..	1995	20.70		..	1995	11.2		..	1995	81.2		..
French Guiana	..	..		..	..	..		..	..	..		..	..	..		..
French Polynesia	..	..		..	..	..		..	..	..		..	..	..		..
Gabon	..	..		..	..	..		..	..	..		..	..	..		..
Gambia, The	..	..		..	..	..		..	..	..		..	..	..		..
Georgia	..	..		..	..	..		..	..	..		..	..	..		..
Germany	..	..		..	1995	20.70		..	1995	14.2		..	1995	83.3		..
Ghana	..	..		..	..	..		..	..	..		..	..	..		..
Greece	..	..		..	1993	13.50		..	1995	8.2		..	1992	70.0		..
Grenada	..	..		..	..	..		..	..	..		..	..	..		..
Guadeloupe	..	..		..	..	..		..	..	..		..	..	..		..
Guam	..	..		..	..	..		..	..	..		..	..	..		..

Table 6. Utilization of Health Services, 1990–95 (*continued*)

Economy	Outpatient visits per capita per year				Inpatient admissions (% of population)				Average number of days per stay				Bed occupancy rate (% of total)			
	Year	Total	Year	Public	Year	Total	Year	Public	Year	Total	Year	Public	Year	Total	Year	Public
Guatemala		..		..		..		..		..		..		..		..
Guinea		..	1994	1.1		..	1994	1.23		..		..		..		..
Guinea-Bissau		..		..		..		..		..		..		..		..
Guyana		..		..		..		..		..		..		..		..
Haiti		..		..		..		..		..		..		..		..
Honduras		..		..		..		..		..		..		..		..
Hong Kong, China	1994	1.0		..	1994	1.50		..		..		..		..		..
Hungary	1994	14.0		..	1995	23.40		..	1995	10.8		..	1995	74.4		..
Iceland	1993	4.8		..	1994	28.00		..	1992	16.8		..	1991	84.0		..
India		..		..		..		..		..		..		..		..
Indonesia		..		..		..		..		..	1993	6.0		..	1993	55.4
Iran, Islamic Republic		..		..		..		..		..		..		..		..
Iraq		..		..		..		..		..		..		..		..
Ireland		..		..	1994	15.40		..	1995	7.2		..	1992	77.0		..
Israel		..		..		..		..		..		..		..		..
Italy		..		..	1994	16.00		..	1995	10.5		..	1994	72.7		..
Jamaica		..	1995	1.1		..		..		..		..		..		..
Japan	1994	16.3		..	1994	8.90		..	1995	45.5		..	1994	83.1		..
Jordan	1994	3.1		..	1994	11.01		..	1994	3.4		..	1994	62.7		..
Kazakhstan		..		..		..		..		..		..		..	1994	74.0
Kenya		..		..		..		..		..		..		..		..
Kiribati		..		..		..		..		..		..		..		..
Korea, Dem. Rep.		..		..		..		..		..		..		..		..
Korea, Rep.	1994	1.8		..	1994	5.70	1994	5.00	1994	19.2	1994	25.8	1995	65.5		..
Kuwait		..		..		..		..		..		..		..		..
Kyrgyz Republic		..		..		..	1994	17.00		..	1994	15.4		..	1994	78.0
Lao PDR		..		..		..		..		..		..		..		..
Latvia		..		..		..		..		..		..		..		..
Lebanon		..		..		..		..		..		..		..		..
Lesotho		..		..		..		..		..		..		..		..
Liberia		..		..		..		..		..		..		..		..
Libya		..		..		..		..		..		..		..		..
Lithuania		..		..		..	1994	20.13		..	1994	16.0		..		..
Luxembourg		..		..	1994	19.40		..	1995	15.3		..	1992	81.4		..
Macao		..		..		..		..		..		..		..		..
Macedonia, FYR		..		..		..		..		..		..		..		..
Madagascar		..		..		..		..		..		..		..		..
Malawi		..	1992	0.9		..	1992	0.02		..	1992	7.0		..	1992	28.0
Malaysia		..	1993	0.7		..	1993	7.26		..	1993	5.4		..	1993	61.7
Maldives		..		..		..		..		..		..		..		..
Mali		..		..		..		..		..		..		..		..
Malta		..		..		..		..		..		..		..		..
Marshall Islands		..	1992	1.0		..		..		..		..		..		..
Martinique		..		..		..		..		..		..		..		..
Mauritania		..		..		..		..		..		..		..		..
Mauritius	1994	3.8	1994	0.3	1994	0.16	1994	0.14		..		..		..		..
Mayotte		..		..		..		..		..		..		..		..
Mexico	1995	1.9		..	1995	5.50		..	1995	4.2		..	1995	65.5		..
Micronesia, Fed. Sts.		..		..		..		..		..		..		..		..
Moldova		..		..		..		..		..		..		..		..
Mongolia		..	1994	5.0		..	1992	22.50		..		..		..	1992	70.0
Montserrat		..		..		..		..		..		..		..		..
Morocco		..		..		..		..		..		..		..		..
Mozambique		..	1991	0.5		..	1991	0.03		..	1991	5.3		..		..
Myanmar		..		..		..		..		..		..		..		..
Namibia		..		..		..		..		..		..		..		..
Nepal		..		..		..		..		..		..		..		..
Netherlands	1995	5.7		..	1995	5.50		..	1995	32.8		..	1995	88.6		..
Netherlands Antilles		..		..		..		..		..		..		..		..
New Caledonia		..		..		..		..		..		..		..		..
New Zealand		..		..	1995	14.10		..	1995	6.9		..	1991	57.3		..
Nicaragua		..		..		..		..		..		..		..		..
Niger		..		..		..		..		..		..		..		..
Nigeria		..		..		..		..		..		..		..		..
Norway	1991	3.8		..	1995	15.00		..	1995	10.0		..	1994	83.0		..
Oman	1990	3.6		..	1990	1.13		..	1990	4.7		..	1990	71.0		..
Pakistan	1994	3.4	1994	1.0		..		..		..		..		..		..
Panama		..		..		..		..		..		..		..		..
Papua New Guinea		..		..		..		..		..		..		..		..
Paraguay		..		..		..		..		..		..		..		..
Peru	1990	1.5		..	1995	0.04		..		..		..		..		..
Philippines		..		..		..	1994	0.23		..		..		..		..
Poland		..		..		..	1994	12.90	1994	11.0		..		..		..
Portugal	1994	3.2		..	1995	11.30		..	1995	9.8		..	1995	71.0		..
Puerto Rico		..		..		..		..		..		..		..		..

Table 6. Utilization of Health Services, 1990–95 (*continued*)

Economy	Outpatient visits per capita per year				Inpatient admissions (% of population)				Average number of days per stay				Bed occupancy rate (% of total)			
	Year	Total	Year	Public	Year	Total	Year	Public	Year	Total	Year	Public	Year	Total	Year	Public
Qatar		..		..		..		..		..		..		..		..
Reunion		..		..		..		..		..		..		..		..
Romania		..		..		..	1994	21.10		..	1994	11.1		..		..
Russian Federation		..		..		..	1993	21.60		..	1993	16.8		..		..
Rwanda		..		..		..		..		..		..		..		..
Samoa		..	1990	1.1		..		..		..		..		..		..
São Tomé and Principe		..		..		..		..		..		..		..		..
Saudi Arabia		..		..		..		..		..		..		..		..
Senegal		..		..		..		..		..		..		..		..
Seychelles	1991	6.0		..		..		..		..		..		..		..
Sierra Leone		..		..		..		..		..		..		..		..
Singapore		..	1994	1.8	1994	11.72	1994	8.80		..		..		..		..
Slovak Republic		..		..		..		..		..	1994	11.4		..		..
Slovenia		..		..		..	1993	15.80		..	1993	10.9		..		..
Solomon Islands	1993	3.4		..		..		..		..		..		..		..
Somalia		..		..		..		..		..		..		..		..
South Africa		..		..		..		..		..		..		..		..
Spain		..		..	1994	10.00		..	1995	11.0		..	1994	76.7		..
Sri Lanka		..		..		..	1994	17.93		..	1994	4.2		..	1994	75.0
St. Kitts and Nevis		..		..		..		..		..		..		..		..
St. Lucia		..		..		..		..		..		..		..		..
St. Vincent and the Grenadines		..		..		..		..		..		..		..		..
Sudan		..		..		..		..		..		..		..		..
Suriname		..		..		..		..		..		..		..		..
Swaziland		..		..		..		..		..		..		..		..
Sweden	1994	3.0		..	1995	18.50		..	1995	7.8		..	1995	82.1		..
Switzerland	1992	11.0		..	1994	15.00		..		..		..	1991	82.6		..
Syrian Arab Republic		..		..		..		..		..		..		..		..
Taiwan, China		..		..		..		..		..		..		..		..
Tajikistan		..		..		..	1992	16.30		..	1992	14.5		..	1991	88.0
Tanzania		..		..		..		..		..		..		..		..
Thailand		..		..		..		..		..		..		..		..
Togo		..		..		..		..		..		..		..		..
Tonga	1991	1.7	1991	1.4		..		..		..		..		..	1992	54.0
Trinidad and Tobago		..		..		..		..		..		..		..		..
Tunisia		..	1990	1.0	1990	8.24		..		..		..		..		..
Turkey	1992	1.0		..	1995	6.30		..	1995	6.4		..	1995	57.4		..
Turkmenistan		..		..		..	1994	16.60		..	1994	15.1		..	1994	64.0
Turks and Caicos Islands		..		..		..		..		..		..		..		..
Uganda		..		..		..		..		..	1991	9.5		..	1991	67.5
Ukraine		..		..		..		..	1994	16.5		..		..		..
United Arab Emirates		..	1992	4.4	1992	11.10	1992	9.76	1993	4.6	1993	4.7	1992	52.0		..
United Kingdom	1993	5.8		..	1995	23.00		..	1995	9.9		..		..		..
United States	1992	5.9		..	1995	12.40		..	1995	8.0		..	1995	66.0		..
Uruguay		..		..		..		..		..		..		..		..
Uzbekistan		..		..		..	1994	19.30		..	1994	14.3		..	1994	87.0
Vanuatu		..	1990	2.3		..		..		..		..		..	1990	28.2
Venezuela		..		..		..		..		..		..		..		..
Vietnam	1993	3.3		..	1993	9.10		..	1993	7.8		..		..		..
Virgin Islands (UK)		..		..		..		..		..		..		..		..
Virgin Islands (US)		..		..		..		..		..		..		..		..
West Bank and Gaza		..		..		..		..		..		..		..		..
Yemen, Rep.		..		..		..		..		..		..		..		..
Yugoslavia, Fed. Republic		..		..		..		..		..		..		..		..
Zambia		..		..		..		..		..		..		..		..
Zimbabwe		..		..		..		..		..		..		..		..

Table 7. Key Development Indicators

Economy	GNP per capita (US$) 1995	Gini coefficient (latest available) 1990–95	Population (thousands) 1995	Population (thousands) 2010	Population growth rate (%) 1980–95	Population growth rate (%) 1995	Population growth rate (%) 1995–2010	Gross secondary school enrollment (% of age group)	Urban population (%) 1995	Crude birth rate (per 1,000 population) 1995	Crude death rate (per 1,000 population) 1995
Afghanistan	..	..	23,481	35,607	2.6	2.8	2.8	..	20	49	21
Albania	670	..	3,260	3,810	1.3	0.0	1.0	..	37	21	6
Algeria	1,600	39	27,959	36,122	2.7	2.2	1.7	61	56	27	6
Angola	410	..	10,772	16,309	2.9	3.1	2.8	14	32	49	19
Anguilla	..	..	..	..	..	..	..	..	..	..	..
Antigua and Barbuda	..	..	65	76	0.4	0.4	1.0	..	35	17	6
Argentina	8,030	..	34,665	40,269	1.4	1.3	1.0	..	88	20	8
Armenia	730	..	3,760	4,262	1.3	1.0	0.8	..	69	14	7
Aruba	..	..	69	..	0.6	0.9	..	..	..	..	..
Australia	18,720	..	18,054	20,371	1.4	1.1	0.8	84	85	15	7
Austria	26,890	..	8,054	8,131	0.4	0.7	0.1	107	56	11	10
Azerbaijan	480	..	7,510	8,725	1.3	0.9	1.0	88	56	21	7
Bahamas, The	11,940	..	276	331	1.8	1.6	1.2	91	87	19	5
Bahrain	7,840	..	577	738	3.6	3.2	1.6	99	90	22	4
Bangladesh	240	28	119,768	149,800	2.2	1.6	1.5	19	18	28	10
Barbados	6,560	..	266	296	0.4	0.8	0.7	..	48	13	9
Belarus	2,070	22	10,339	10,477	0.5	0.2	0.1	92	71	11	12
Belgium	24,710	..	10,146	10,236	0.2	0.4	0.1	103	97	12	11
Belize	..	..	216	296	2.6	2.6	2.1	38	47	33	5
Benin	370	..	5,475	8,098	3.1	2.9	2.6	12	42	44	15
Bermuda	..	..	63	..	1.0	0.8	..	..	..	..	..
Bhutan	420	..	695	1,238	..	..	3.8	..	..	..	..
Bolivia	800	42	7,414	10,217	2.2	2.4	2.1	..	58	35	10
Bosnia and Herzegovina	..	..	4,383	4,762	0.5	0.0	0.6	..	49	..	..
Botswana	3,020	..	1,450	1,872	3.2	2.4	1.7	19	31	35	11
Brazil	3,640	63	159,222	189,875	1.8	1.4	1.2	43	78	21	7
Brunei	25,160	..	285	355	2.6	1.9	1.5	71	59	23	4
Bulgaria	1,330	31	8,409	7,986	−0.3	−0.7	−0.3	72	71	10	13
Burkina Faso	230	..	10,377	15,332	2.7	2.8	2.6	8	27	46	18
Burundi	160	..	6,264	9,181	2.8	2.6	2.5	7	8	44	18
Cambodia	270	..	10,024	13,526	2.9	2.8	2.0	..	21	41	13
Cameroon	650	..	13,288	20,488	2.8	2.9	2.9	32	45	41	11
Canada	19,380	..	29,606	32,251	1.2	1.3	0.6	88	77	13	7
Cape Verde	960	..	380	507	1.8	2.2	1.9	..	54	34	8
Cayman Islands	..	..	..	..	..	..	..	..	..	..	..
Central African Republic	340	..	3,275	4,409	2.3	2.2	2.0	..	39	39	17
Chad	180	..	6,448	9,262	2.4	2.5	2.4	9	21	43	18
Channel Islands	..	..	142	140	0.6	−0.1	−0.1	..	29	12	10
Chile	4,160	57	14,225	16,856	1.6	1.5	1.1	70	86	20	6
China	620	42	1,203,324	1,346,656	1.4	1.1	0.8	52	30	17	7
Colombia	1,910	51	36,813	44,956	1.8	1.8	1.3	62	73	24	7
Comoros	470	..	499	774	2.7	2.9	2.9	19	28	43	12
Congo, Dem. Rep.	120	..	43,848	71,958	3.2	3.2	3.3	24	29	..	..
Congo, Rep.	680	..	2,633	3,913	3.0	2.9	2.6	..	59	47	16
Costa Rica	2,610	46	3,399	4,256	2.7	2.4	1.5	47	50	25	4
Côte d'Ivoire	660	37	13,978	19,437	3.6	3.0	2.2	25	44	37	12
Croatia	3,250	..	4,778	4,749	0.3	0.0	0.0	83	64	11	11
Cuba	..	..	11,011	11,976	0.8	0.6	0.6	77	76	14	7
Cyprus	..	..	734	835	1.2	1.4	0.9	95	54	16	7
Czech Republic	3,870	27	10,332	10,382	0.1	0.1	0.0	86	65	10	11
Denmark	29,890	..	5,220	5,294	0.1	0.3	0.1	114	85	13	12
Djibouti	..	..	634	993	5.4	4.9	3.0	12	83	46	16
Dominica	2,990	..	73	89	0.0	0.3	1.3	..	..	23	6
Dominican Republic	1,460	51	7,822	9,464	2.1	1.9	1.3	..	65	25	5
Ecuador	1,390	47	11,477	14,841	2.4	2.2	1.7	55	58	27	6
Egypt, Arab Rep.	790	32	57,800	73,308	2.3	1.9	1.6	76	45	27	8
El Salvador	1,610	..	5,623	7,586	1.4	2.3	2.0	29	45	31	6
Equatorial Guinea	380	..	400	585	4.1	2.8	2.5	..	42	44	17
Eritrea	..	..	3,574	5,449	..	2.6	2.8	14	17	43	16
Estonia	2,860	40	1,487	1,375	0.0	−1.3	−0.5	92	73	10	14
Ethiopia	100	..	56,404	85,779	2.7	2.7	2.8	11	13	47	17
Fiji	2,440	..	775	887	1.3	1.1	0.9	64	41	23	5
Finland	20,580	..	5,110	5,291	0.4	0.5	0.2	119	63	13	10
France	24,990	..	58,060	60,323	0.5	0.4	0.3	106	73	12	9
French Guiana	..	..	..	..	..	..	..	..	..	..	..
French Polynesia	..	..	225	299	2.4	2.7	1.9	77	..	27	5
Gabon	3,490	..	1,077	1,525	3.0	2.5	2.3	..	50	39	15
Gambia, The	320	..	1,113	1,530	3.7	3.6	2.1	19	26	41	18
Georgia	440	..	5,400	5,504	0.4	−0.3	0.1	..	58	11	9
Germany	27,510	..	81,869	82,029	0.3	0.6	0.0	101	87	9	11
Ghana	390	34	17,075	24,619	3.1	2.7	2.4	36	36	37	10
Greece	8,210	..	10,467	10,767	0.5	0.5	0.2	..	65	10	9
Grenada	2,980	..	91	95	0.1	..	0.3	..	..	..	..
Guadeloupe	..	..	424	511	1.7	1.5	1.2	..	51	19	6
Guam	..	..	149	181	2.2	2.3	1.3	..	38	22	4

37

Table 7. Key Development Indicators (*continued*)

Economy	GNP per capita (US$) 1995	Gini coefficient (latest available) 1990–95	Population (thousands) 1995	Population (thousands) 2010	Population growth rate (%) 1980–95	Population growth rate (%) 1995	Population growth rate (%) 1995–2010	Gross secondary school enrollment (% of age group)	Urban population (%) 1995	Crude birth rate (per 1,000 population) 1995	Crude death rate (per 1,000 population) 1995
Guatemala	1,340	60	10,621	15,434	2.9	2.9	2.5	24	42	36	7
Guinea	550	47	6,591	10,055	2.6	2.7	2.8	12	30	48	20
Guinea-Bissau	250	56	1,070	1,461	1.9	2.1	2.1	..	22	45	25
Guyana	590	..	835	977	0.6	1.0	1.0	..	36	23	8
Haiti	250	..	7,168	8,771	1.9	2.1	1.3	..	32	35	12
Honduras	600	53	5,924	8,590	3.2	3.0	2.5	32	48	36	6
Hong Kong, China	22,990	..	6,190	6,420	1.4	1.8	0.2	..	95	11	5
Hungary	4,120	27	10,229	9,959	–0.3	–0.3	–0.2	81	65	11	14
Iceland	24,950	..	268	301	1.1	1.0	0.8	103	92	16	7
India	340	34	929,358	1,127,143	2.0	1.7	1.3	..	27	26	9
Indonesia	980	32	193,277	234,519	1.8	1.6	1.3	43	34	23	8
Iran, Islamic Republic	..	..	64,120	91,403	3.3	2.7	2.4	66	59	32	6
Iraq	..	..	20,097	31,397	2.9	2.1	3.0	44	75	38	9
Ireland	14,710	..	3,586	3,962	0.4	0.4	0.7	105	58	14	9
Israel	15,920	..	5,521	6,783	2.4	2.7	1.4	87	..	20	6
Italy	19,020	..	57,204	56,497	0.1	0.2	–0.1	81	67	9	10
Jamaica	1,510	41	2,522	2,924	1.1	1.0	1.0	66	55	22	6
Japan	39,640	..	125,213	127,946	0.5	0.3	0.1	96	78	10	7
Jordan	1,510	43	4,212	6,034	4.4	4.3	2.4	..	71	32	5
Kazakhstan	1,330	33	16,606	18,470	0.7	–0.4	0.7	..	60	18	9
Kenya	280	58	26,688	37,132	3.2	2.6	2.2	25	28	35	9
Kiribati	920	..	79	98	2.0	1.9	1.4	..	..	28	9
Korea, Dem. Rep.	..	..	23,867	28,888	1.8	1.8	1.3	..	61	22	6
Korea, Rep.	9,700	..	44,851	50,376	1.1	0.9	0.8	93	81	16	6
Kuwait	17,390	..	1,664	2,464	1.3	5.0	2.6	..	97	22	3
Kyrgyz Republic	700	..	4,515	5,309	1.5	0.3	1.1	..	39	25	8
Lao PDR	350	30	4,882	7,408	2.8	3.0	2.8	25	22	44	15
Latvia	2,270	27	2,516	2,264	–0.1	–1.4	–0.7	87	73	9	16
Lebanon	2,660	..	4,005	4,903	2.3	1.9	1.3	76	87	26	8
Lesotho	770	56	1,980	2,704	2.5	2.1	2.1	26	23	33	11
Liberia	..	..	2,733	4,238	2.5	2.4	2.9	..	45	47	20
Libya	..	..	5,407	8,796	3.8	3.5	3.2	97	86	41	8
Lithuania	1,900	34	3,715	3,658	0.6	–0.2	–0.1	78	72	11	12
Luxembourg	41,210	..	410	437	0.8	1.4	0.4	..	89	13	9
Macao	..	..	450	528	3.0	3.4	1.1	..	99	19	5
Macedonia, FYR	860	..	2,119	2,380	0.8	1.0	0.8	54	60	16	7
Madagascar	230	43	13,651	20,926	3.0	3.1	2.8	18	27	42	11
Malawi	170	..	9,757	13,961	3.1	2.7	2.4	4	14	47	20
Malaysia	3,890	48	20,140	26,323	2.5	2.4	1.8	59	54	27	5
Maldives	990	..	253	409	3.1	3.2	3.2	49	33	41	8
Mali	250	..	9,788	15,314	2.6	2.9	3.0	9	27	50	17
Malta	..	..	372	409	0.1	1.0	0.6	88	89	13	7
Marshall Islands	..	..	..	..	..	..	..	..	..	..	..
Martinique	..	..	380	432	1.0	1.1	0.9	..	78	17	7
Mauritania	460	42	2,274	3,223	2.6	2.5	2.3	15	54	39	14
Mauritius	3,380	..	1,128	1,312	1.0	1.4	1.0	59	41	19	7
Mayotte	..	..	..	..	..	..	..	..	..	..	..
Mexico	3,320	50	91,831	114,244	2.1	1.9	1.5	58	75	26	5
Micronesia, Fed. Sts.	2,010	..	107	154	2.7	2.2	2.4	..	28	33	7
Moldova	..	34	4,344	4,552	0.5	–0.1	0.3	69	52	14	11
Mongolia	310	..	2,461	3,244	2.6	2.1	1.8	82	61	27	7
Montserrat	..	..	12	..	0.4	0.4	..	..	14	20	10
Morocco	1,110	39	26,562	33,974	2.1	2.0	1.6	35	48	27	7
Mozambique	80	..	17,423	25,352	1.9	2.9	2.4	7	34	44	18
Myanmar	..	..	45,106	57,104	1.9	1.7	1.6	..	26	28	10
Namibia	2,000	..	1,545	2,180	2.7	2.7	2.3	55	37	37	12
Nepal	200	37	21,456	29,914	2.5	2.5	2.2	21	14	37	12
Netherlands	24,000	..	15,460	16,063	0.6	0.6	0.3	93	89	12	9
Netherlands Antilles	..	..	200	231	0.9	1.1	1.0	..	70	19	6
New Caledonia	..	..	185	226	2.0	1.9	1.3	85	62	21	6
New Zealand	14,340	..	3,601	4,086	1.0	1.4	0.8	104	86	16	8
Nicaragua	380	50	4,375	6,236	3.0	3.1	2.4	41	63	34	6
Niger	220	36	9,028	14,575	3.3	3.3	3.2	7	23	52	19
Nigeria	260	38	111,273	164,073	3.0	2.9	2.6	29	39	42	14
Norway	31,250	..	4,354	4,566	0.4	0.5	0.3	116	73	14	10
Oman	4,820	..	2,196	3,884	4.6	5.5	3.8	61	13	44	4
Pakistan	460	31	129,905	189,852	3.0	2.9	2.5	..	35	38	9
Panama	2,750	57	2,631	3,218	2.0	1.6	1.3	64	55	23	5
Papua New Guinea	1,160	..	4,302	5,789	2.2	2.3	2.0	12	16	33	10
Paraguay	1,690	..	4,828	6,644	2.9	2.7	2.1	37	53	31	5
Peru	2,310	45	23,819	30,470	2.1	2.0	1.6	65	72	26	7
Philippines	1,050	41	68,595	90,101	2.3	2.2	1.8	79	54	29	7
Poland	2,790	27	38,612	40,286	0.5	0.2	0.3	79	65	13	10
Portugal	9,740	..	9,927	10,010	0.1	0.1	0.1	81	36	11	10
Puerto Rico	..	..	3,717	4,215	1.0	1.1	0.8	..	73	17	8

Table 7. Key Development Indicators (*continued*)

Economy	GNP per capita (US$) 1995	Gini coefficient (latest available) 1990–95	Population (thousands) 1995	Population (thousands) 2010	Population growth rate (%) 1980–95	Population growth rate (%) 1995	Population growth rate (%) 1995–2010	Gross secondary school enrollment (% of age group)	Urban population (%) 1995	Crude birth rate (per 1,000 population) 1995	Crude death rate (per 1,000 population) 1995
Qatar	11,600	..	642	918	6.9	5.8	2.4	83	91	21	4
Reunion	..	..	653	782	1.7	1.7	1.2	..	68	20	5
Romania	1,480	26	22,692	22,462	0.1	–0.5	–0.1	82	55	11	12
Russian Federation	2,240	50	148,195	144,952	0.4	–0.1	–0.1	88	73	9	15
Rwanda	180	29	6,400	10,764	1.4	–2.8	3.5	10	6	41	23
Samoa	1,120	..	165	204	0.4	0.6	1.4	..	21	33	7
São Tomé and Principe	350	..	129	183	2.1	2.5	2.3	..	47	35	8
Saudi Arabia	6,810	..	18,979	30,941	4.7	3.8	3.3	29	80	36	5
Senegal	600	54	8,468	12,374	2.8	2.6	2.5	11	42	40	14
Seychelles	6,620	..	74	93	1.0	1.6	1.6	..	65	22	7
Sierra Leone	180	..	4,195	6,270	1.7	0.8	2.7	..	36	48	30
Singapore	26,730	..	2,987	3,478	1.8	1.9	1.0	84	100	16	5
Slovak Republic	2,950	20	5,369	5,562	0.5	0.4	0.2	89	59	12	10
Slovenia	8,200	28	1,992	1,986	0.3	–0.1	0.0	85	64	10	10
Solomon Islands	910	..	375	559	3.2	3.0	2.7	17	17	37	8
Somalia	..	..	9,491	15,399	2.3	4.1	3.2	..	26	49	18
South Africa	3,160	58	36,956	53,492	2.1	1.8	1.4	77	51	30	8
Spain	13,580	..	39,199	39,423	0.3	0.2	0.0	113	76	10	9
Sri Lanka	700	30	18,114	21,477	1.4	1.2	1.1	74	22	20	6
St. Kitts and Nevis	5,170	..	41	46	–0.5	–0.5	0.8	..	46	20	12
St. Lucia	3,370	..	158	194	1.6	0.9	1.4	..	46	28	6
St. Vincent and the Grenadines	2,280	..	111	128	0.8	0.7	1.0	..	47	22	7
Sudan	..	..	26,707	37,413	2.4	2.1	2.2	20	25	35	12
Suriname	880	..	410	457	0.9	0.4	0.7	..	50	24	6
Swaziland	1,170	..	900	1,321	3.1	2.5	2.6	51	31	34	9
Sweden	23,750	..	8,830	9,143	0.4	0.6	0.2	99	83	13	10
Switzerland	40,630	..	7,039	7,287	0.7	0.9	0.2	91	61	12	9
Syrian Arab Republic	1,120	..	14,112	21,144	3.2	3.0	2.7	47	52	39	5
Taiwan, China	12,790	..	21,137	23,571	1.2	0.8	0.7	..	..	15	6
Tajikistan	340	..	5,836	7,721	2.6	1.6	1.9	100	32	28	7
Tanzania	120	38	29,646	43,775	3.1	3.0	2.6	5	24	43	14
Thailand	2,740	46	58,242	64,725	1.5	0.9	0.7	37	20	17	6
Togo	310	..	4,085	6,148	3.0	2.9	2.7	27	31	44	15
Tonga	1,630	..	104	135	0.7	3.1	1.7	..	41	28	6
Trinidad and Tobago	3,770	..	1,287	1,487	1.2	0.8	1.0	76	67	19	6
Tunisia	1,820	40	8,987	11,207	2.3	1.8	1.5	52	57	24	6
Turkey	2,780	..	61,058	74,996	2.1	1.6	1.4	61	69	23	7
Turkmenistan	920	36	4,508	6,400	3.0	4.5	2.3	..	45	31	7
Turks and Caicos Islands	..	..	..	..	..	..	..	..	..	..	..
Uganda	240	41	19,168	28,100	2.7	3.2	2.6	13	13	49	19
Ukraine	1,630	26	51,550	49,763	0.2	–0.2	–0.2	80	70	10	14
United Arab Emirates	17,400	..	2,460	3,397	5.7	5.0	2.2	89	84	20	3
United Kingdom	18,700	..	58,533	60,149	0.3	0.3	0.2	92	89	13	11
United States	26,980	..	263,119	297,205	1.0	1.0	0.8	97	76	15	8
Uruguay	5,170	..	3,184	3,491	0.6	0.6	0.6	81	90	17	10
Uzbekistan	970	..	22,771	30,582	2.4	2.1	2.0	..	41	29	6
Vanuatu	1,200	..	169	241	2.6	2.7	2.4	20	..	35	7
Venezuela	3,020	54	21,671	27,849	2.5	2.3	1.7	35	93	25	5
Vietnam	..	36	73,475	93,360	2.1	2.0	1.6	35	21	26	7
Virgin Islands (UK)	..	..	..	..	..	..	..	..	..	..	..
Virgin Islands (US)	..	..	99	96	0.1	–0.5	–0.2	..	49	20	5
West Bank and Gaza	..	..	..	..	..	..	..	..	..	..	..
Yemen, Rep.	260	..	15,272	25,222	3.9	3.2	3.3	..	34	48	13
Yugoslavia, Fed. Republic	..	..	10,518	10,863	0.7	0.1	0.2	65	57	14	10
Zambia	400	46	8,978	12,354	3.0	2.9	2.1	..	43	45	17
Zimbabwe	540	57	11,011	13,959	3.0	2.4	1.6	45	32	31	9
World	5,120	..	5,673,000	6,850,000	1.6	1.5	1.3	57	40	23	9
Low-income	440	..	3,180,000	3,971,000	1.9	1.7	1.5	..	21	26	10
Excluding China and India	310	..	1,050,000	1,479,000	2.6	2.4	2.3	22	21	37	13
Middle-income	2,450	..	1,591,000	1,916,000	1.7	1.6	1.2	61	52	22	8
Low- and middle-income	1,100	..	4,771,000	5,887,000	1.9	1.7	1.4	52	32	25	9
East Asia and Pacific	800	..	1,706,000	1,974,000	1.5	1.3	1.0	52	21	19	7
Europe and Central Asia	2,130	..	488,000	511,000	0.7	0.3	0.3	86	58	14	11
Latin America and the Caribbean	3,310	..	478,000	587,000	1.9	1.7	1.4	59	65	24	7
Middle East and North Africa	1,760	..	272,000	383,000	3.0	2.5	2.3	51	48	32	7
South Asia	350	..	1,243,000	1,572,000	2.1	1.9	1.6	..	22	28	9
Sub-Saharan Africa	510	..	583,000	860,000	2.8	2.6	2.6	24	23	41	15
High-income	24,790	..	902,000	963,000	0.7	0.7	0.4	97	75	13	8

Table 8. Child Mortality, 1960–95

	Mortaility rate per 1,000 live births									
	Infants					Children under five				
Economy	1960	1970	1980	1990	1995	1960	1970	1980	1990	1995
Afghanistan	215	199	183	168	159	366	..	..	..	237
Albania	83	68	48	28	31	..	..	..	..	37
Algeria	168	141	100	46	34	255	192	139	..	42
Angola	208	180	155	131	124	..	..	..	..	209
Anguilla	..	..	..	..	..	..	..	..	..	..
Antigua and Barbuda	..	..	32	21	19	..	..	..	..	23
Argentina	60	53	36	26	22	72	71	38	28	27
Armenia	..	..	26	19	16	..	..	..	..	24
Aruba	..	..	..	..	..	..	..	..	..	..
Australia	20	18	11	8	6	..	..	..	..	8
Austria	38	26	14	8	6	..	..	..	..	7
Azerbaijan	..	..	30	23	25	..	..	..	..	31
Bahamas, The	52	35	30	28	15	..	..	..	..	18
Bahrain	130	67	44	24	19	..	..	..	..	23
Bangladesh	156	140	133	98	80	247	237	207	139	115
Barbados	74	40	22	12	13	..	..	..	..	12
Belarus	..	..	16	12	13	..	..	..	..	20
Belgium	31	21	12	8	8	..	..	..	..	10
Belize	..	..	..	46	37	..	..	..	..	46
Benin	185	156	123	103	96	..	256	205	..	156
Bermuda	..	..	..	8	..	..	..	..	..	..
Bhutan	..	..	..	..	..	..	..	..	..	175
Bolivia	167	154	120	83	70	255	243	171	124	96
Bosnia and Herzegovina	105	62	32	19	..	..	..	..	..	..
Botswana	116	97	70	56	56	173	146	80	..	74
Brazil	116	96	72	51	45	177	135	86	..	57
Brunei	63	58	19	10	9	..	..	..	..	11
Bulgaria	45	27	20	15	15	..	..	..	..	19
Burkina Faso	186	143	122	106	100	314	278	241	197	164
Burundi	153	139	122	108	99	250	233	195	168	162
Cambodia	146	156	212	123	109	..	..	..	..	158
Cameroon	163	128	95	68	57	..	215	172	127	86
Canada	27	19	10	7	6	..	..	..	..	8
Cape Verde	110	87	68	54	47	..	..	..	..	68
Cayman Islands	..	..	..	..	..	..	..	..	..	..
Central African Republic	175	141	118	102	98	343	238	193	..	160
Chad	195	173	149	128	118	..	..	206	..	197
Channel Islands	24	19	11	8	7	..	..	..	..	9
Chile	114	79	35	17	12	155	97	37	19	15
China	132	69	42	38	35	173	115	60	45	43
Colombia	99	75	47	31	26	122	113	58	..	31
Comoros	..	..	..	103	89	..	..	..	..	143
Congo, Dem. Rep.	153	132	112	..	..	..	245	..	..	144
Congo, Rep.	142	103	89	87	90	209	..	..	..	144
Costa Rica	74	62	20	15	13	124	85	29	..	16
Côte d'Ivoire	166	136	109	92	86	..	237	157	..	138
Croatia	..	..	21	11	16	..	..	..	..	18
Cuba	35	39	20	11	9	49	43	22	12	10
Cyprus	30	29	18	11	8	..	..	..	..	11
Czech Republic	22	21	17	11	8	..	..	..	..	10
Denmark	22	14	8	8	6	..	..	..	..	7
Djibouti	186	160	138	118	109	..	..	..	..	181
Dominica	..	..	13	19	17	..	..	..	..	21
Dominican Republic	125	100	78	49	38	149	127	92	58	44
Ecuador	124	101	69	47	37	178	140	98	50	45
Egypt, Arab Rep.	179	160	122	71	57	..	235	175	95	76
El Salvador	130	105	82	48	37	191	161	125	54	42
Equatorial Guinea	188	165	143	122	112	..	..	..	..	185
Eritrea	..	..	..	135	132	..	..	..	..	196
Estonia	36	20	17	12	14	..	..	..	..	16
Ethiopia	175	159	154	126	113	..	239	213	..	188
Fiji	71	50	34	25	21	..	..	..	..	25
Finland	22	14	8	6	5	..	..	..	..	5
France	27	18	10	7	6	..	..	..	..	9
French Guiana	..	..	..	..	..	..	..	..	..	..
French Polynesia	..	..	..	25	17	..	..	..	..	24
Gabon	171	140	117	99	90	..	..	..	..	145
Gambia, The	213	186	161	137	127	..	..	..	..	213
Georgia	..	..	25	16	18	..	..	..	..	21
Germany	35	23	12	7	6	..	..	..	..	7
Ghana	132	112	100	84	74	214	187	157	127	116
Greece	40	30	18	10	8	..	..	..	..	10
Grenada	..	..	..	..	..	..	..	..	..	32
Guadeloupe	50	46	20	13	11	..	..	..	..	14
Guam	27	22	16	11	9	..	..	..	..	12

Table 8. Child Mortality, 1960–95 (*continued*)

	Infants					Children under five				
Economy	*1960*	*1970*	*1980*	*1990*	*1995*	*1960*	*1970*	*1980*	*1990*	*1995*
Guatemala	125	102	76	55	45	204	168	140	73	58
Guinea	203	182	162	140	129	..	..	..	..	220
Guinea-Bissau	201	186	170	146	137	..	..	..	..	233
Guyana	100	81	68	65	61	..	..	..	..	82
Haiti	182	143	124	88	73	..	221	200	148	101
Honduras	160	113	70	50	46	204	170	101	..	59
Hong Kong, China	44	20	11	6	5	55	23	12	7	6
Hungary	48	36	23	15	11	..	..	..	..	14
Iceland	13	13	8	6	4	..	..	..	..	6
India	165	139	119	86	69	242	202	173	110	95
Indonesia	139	119	93	65	52	216	172	124	95	75
Iran, Islamic Rep.	169	134	95	55	46	281	191	130	..	59
Iraq	139	104	81	96	111	161	123	93	..	145
Ireland	29	20	11	8	6	..	..	..	..	7
Israel	31	25	15	10	8	38	28	19	10	9
Italy	44	30	15	8	7	..	..	..	..	8
Jamaica	63	44	22	16	13	74	64	34	..	15
Japan	30	13	8	5	4	..	..	..	..	6
Jordan	..	..	41	34	31	139	107	64	36	33
Kazakhstan	..	..	33	26	27	..	..	..	..	35
Kenya	124	103	74	62	59	205	156	115	97	90
Kiribati	..	107	..	63	56	..	..	..	..	75
Korea, Dem. Rep.	90	53	33	28	40	..	..	..	..	45
Korea, Rep.	85	48	27	13	10	127	55	18	..	14
Kuwait	89	49	28	14	11	126	54	33	..	14
Kyrgyz Republic	..	..	43	30	30	..	..	..	..	42
Lao PDR	155	146	129	104	92	..	..	..	..	147
Latvia	35	22	21	14	16	..	..	..	..	20
Lebanon	68	50	48	37	32	84	..	..	..	40
Lesotho	149	135	111	86	77	203	190	..	..	121
Liberia	184	177	160	171	177	284	270	235	..	239
Libya	160	124	102	75	45	270	..	..	..	55
Lithuania	55	25	20	13	14	..	..	..	..	19
Luxembourg	32	25	12	7	6	..	..	..	..	9
Macao	..	..	..	10	7	..	..	..	..	9
Macedonia, FYR	..	..	54	32	23	..	..	..	..	31
Madagascar	220	184	140	103	90	186	..	175	170	127
Malawi	207	194	170	136	133	360	347	271	233	225
Malaysia	73	46	31	15	12	..	..	..	..	14
Maldives	160	129	100	71	53	..	..	..	..	70
Mali	210	205	186	135	124	..	..	291	..	192
Malta	38	28	15	9	9	..	..	..	..	11
Marshall Islands	..	..	..	..	..	..	..	..	..	..
Martinique	52	39	18	10	8	..	..	..	..	12
Mauritania	177	150	121	106	97	..	..	..	..	158
Mauritius	70	61	33	21	16	88	83	38	24	20
Mayotte	..	..	..	..	..	..	..	..	..	..
Mexico	92	74	52	38	33	134	111	76	47	41
Micronesia, Fed. Sts.	..	..	..	40	33	..	..	..	..	40
Moldova	..	..	35	19	22	..	..	..	..	26
Mongolia	128	103	83	64	56	..	..	..	..	74
Montserrat	..	..	36	30	25	..	..	..	..	31
Morocco	163	130	101	65	56	..	187	147	76	75
Mozambique	190	172	148	122	114	..	281	285	..	190
Myanmar	158	129	110	97	84	..	179	134	..	119
Namibia	146	119	91	66	62	..	..	108	86	78
Nepal	195	168	134	103	92	300	232	179	..	131
Netherlands	18	13	9	7	6	..	..	..	..	8
Netherlands Antilles	..	..	..	11	11	..	..	..	..	14
New Caledonia	..	..	..	19	16	..	..	..	..	19
New Zealand	23	17	13	8	7	..	..	..	..	9
Nicaragua	140	108	92	62	47	193	165	120	..	61
Niger	191	171	152	130	120	..	..	300	321	..
Nigeria	190	141	100	86	81	..	..	196	190	176
Norway	19	13	8	7	5	..	..	..	..	8
Oman	214	129	43	23	18	..	..	..	..	22
Pakistan	163	143	125	100	91	226	183	161	138	127
Panama	69	48	33	27	23	88	68	47	..	28
Papua New Guinea	165	115	68	64	65	204	..	..	..	95
Paraguay	66	56	50	45	41	92	76	59	..	52
Peru	142	108	81	54	48	234	178	126	73	62
Philippines	80	67	53	44	40	107	82	69	..	53
Poland	56	33	21	16	14	..	..	..	..	16
Portugal	78	56	24	11	7	..	..	..	..	11
Puerto Rico	43	29	19	14	11	55	34	22	15	15

Table 8. Child Mortality, 1960–95 (continued)

	Mortality rate per 1,000 live births									
	Infants					Children under five				
Economy	1960	1970	1980	1990	1995	1960	1970	1980	1990	1995
Qatar	145	71	42	22	19	..	..	..	..	22
Reunion	99	57	18	8	8	..	..	..	..	10
Romania	76	49	29	27	23	..	..	..	..	29
Russian Federation	..	..	22	17	18	..	..	..	..	21
Rwanda	150	143	129	131	135	206	209	218	..	200
Samoa	..	..	..	28	23	..	..	..	..	27
São Tomé and Principe	..	..	83	70	61	..	..	..	..	78
Saudi Arabia	170	123	67	33	21	..	..	..	..	31
Senegal	172	138	92	72	63	297	279	218	138	97
Seychelles	..	..	..	17	15	..	..	..	..	19
Sierra Leone	219	199	191	188	182	390	360	335	..	236
Singapore	35	20	12	7	4	47	25	13	7	6
Slovak Republic	34	25	21	12	11	..	..	..	..	15
Slovenia	37	25	16	8	7	..	..	..	..	8
Solomon Islands	..	..	67	48	41	..	..	..	..	52
Somalia	175	159	146	132	129	..	..	..	..	218
South Africa	89	80	68	56	51	..	..	..	..	67
Spain	44	28	12	8	7	..	..	..	..	9
Sri Lanka	71	55	36	19	16	133	100	48	..	19
St. Kitts and Nevis	..	..	..	26	31	..	..	..	..	38
St. Lucia	..	..	..	20	17	..	..	..	..	21
St. Vincent and the Grenadines	..	..	..	21	19	..	..	..	..	22
Sudan	160	120	95	85	78	204	176	132	..	109
Suriname	70	54	47	39	34	..	..	..	..	41
Swaziland	152	140	114	81	70	..	..	..	..	96
Sweden	17	11	7	6	4	..	..	..	..	5
Switzerland	21	15	9	7	6	..	..	..	..	7
Syrian Arab Republic	135	98	58	40	33	200	128	74	42	40
Taiwan, China	..	..	..	9	6	..	..	..	..	7
Tajikistan	..	..	58	41	42	..	..	..	..	61
Tanzania	147	130	106	89	83	240	218	176	161	133
Thailand	103	75	50	38	35	148	102	58	..	42
Togo	182	135	111	93	89	267	..	175	..	128
Tonga	..	..	52	24	19	..	..	..	..	23
Trinidad and Tobago	62	53	36	19	14	61	55	39	24	18
Tunisia	159	124	73	46	40	254	201	100	..	50
Turkey	190	146	111	67	49	219	201	133	70	63
Turkmenistan	..	..	54	45	46	..	..	..	..	65
Turks and Caicos Islands	..	..	..	..	..	..	..	..	..	..
Uganda	133	110	116	106	98	224	..	180	..	160
Ukraine	41	23	17	13	15	..	..	..	..	21
United Arab Emirates	145	87	58	21	16	223	83	..	26	19
United Kingdom	23	19	12	8	6	..	..	..	..	7
United States	26	20	13	9	8	..	..	..	..	10
Uruguay	51	47	38	22	18	56	56	43	24	21
Uzbekistan	..	..	47	35	30	..	..	..	..	48
Vanuatu	..	..	..	59	42	..	..	..	..	51
Venezuela	81	55	37	25	23	75	62	42	26	25
Vietnam	156	108	57	46	41	..	..	60	..	49
Virgin Islands (UK)	..	..	..	..	..	..	..	..	..	..
Virgin Islands (US)	33		22	20	19	..	..	..	..	23
West Bank and Gaza	..	..	..	..	..	..	..	..	..	..
Yemen, Rep.	214	188	144	111	101	..	..	198	..	145
Yugoslavia, Fed. Rep.	87	54	36	25	18	..	..	..	..	22
Zambia	135	108	91	109	109	213	181	149	188	180
Zimbabwe	110	97	83	60	55	159	137	107	80	83
World	128	98	82	62	55	..	..	..	..	81
Low-income	153	114	98	77	69	..	..	..	..	104
Excluding China and India	167	140	117	97	89	..	..	..	..	143
Middle-income	120	94	69	46	39	..	..	..	..	53
Low- and middle-income	143	108	90	68	60	..	..	..	..	88
East Asia and Pacific	131	80	56	45	40	..	..	..	..	53
Europe and Central Asia	95	71	50	30	26	..	..	..	..	35
Latin America and the Caribbean	105	85	62	43	37	..	..	..	..	47
Middle East and North Africa	165	137	99	62	54	..	..	..	..	72
South Asia	164	140	122	90	75	..	..	..	..	106
Sub-Saharan Africa	170	138	115	99	92	..	..	..	..	157
High-income	35	26	13	8	7	..	..	..	..	9

Table 9. Life Expectancy at Birth, 1960–95

	Life expectancy at birth (years)											
	Male						Female					
Economy	1960	1970	1980	1990	1995	% change 1960–95	1960	1970	1980	1990	1995	% change 1960–95
Afghanistan	33	37	40	42	44	32	34	37	41	43	45	34
Albania	61	66	67	69	70	14	63	68	72	75	76	21
Algeria	46	52	58	66	68	48	48	54	60	69	71	48
Angola	32	36	39	44	45	42	35	39	43	47	48	39
Anguilla	..	..	..	..	..	..	..	..	..	..	..	..
Antigua and Barbuda	61	65	..	71	72	19	64	69	..	76	78	21
Argentina	62	63	66	68	69	11	68	70	73	75	76	12
Armenia	65	69	70	67	68	5	71	75	76	73	74	5
Aruba	..	..	..	..	..	..	..	..	..	..	..	..
Australia	68	68	71	73	74	9	74	75	78	80	80	9
Austria	66	67	69	72	74	13	72	74	76	79	80	12
Azerbaijan	60	64	64	67	66	9	68	72	72	75	75	10
Bahamas, The	61	63	64	68	70	15	66	69	72	75	77	17
Bahrain	54	60	66	69	70	31	57	64	70	74	75	31
Bangladesh	41	45	49	55	57	39	38	43	48	55	58	52
Barbados	62	66	70	72	73	18	67	71	75	77	78	17
Belarus	64	68	66	66	64	0	73	76	76	76	75	4
Belgium	67	68	70	73	73	9	73	75	77	79	80	9
Belize	..	57	..	72	73	..	..	61	..	74	76	..
Benin	38	43	45	49	49	29	39	45	49	52	52	32
Bermuda	..	..	..	..	..	..	..	..	..	..	..	..
Bhutan	..	..	..	..	..	..	..	..	..	..	..	..
Bolivia	41	44	50	56	59	45	45	48	54	60	62	39
Bosnia and Herzegovina	59	64	68	69	..	..	62	68	73	74	..	..
Botswana	45	50	56	56	51	13	48	53	60	59	54	12
Brazil	53	57	60	62	63	19	57	61	65	69	71	25
Brunei	62	65	69	72	73	18	63	68	73	76	78	24
Bulgaria	67	69	69	68	68	2	70	74	74	75	75	6
Burkina Faso	35	39	43	45	45	30	37	41	45	47	47	26
Burundi	40	42	45	45	44	12	43	45	49	48	47	11
Cambodia	41	42	38	49	51	25	44	44	40	52	54	23
Cameroon	38	43	48	53	55	46	41	46	51	56	58	43
Canada	68	69	71	74	75	11	74	76	78	81	81	10
Cape Verde	51	55	59	63	65	28	54	58	62	65	67	24
Cayman Islands	..	..	..	..	..	..	..	..	..	..	..	..
Central African Republic	36	40	43	46	46	28	41	45	48	51	51	24
Chad	33	37	40	45	46	40	36	40	44	48	50	37
Channel Islands	..	..	..	73	74	..	..	..	..	80	82	..
Chile	55	59	66	71	72	32	60	65	72	77	78	30
China	35	61	..	67	68	93	38	62	..	70	71	89
Colombia	55	59	63	66	67	22	58	63	68	72	73	25
Comoros	42	46	50	52	54	28	43	47	51	55	57	34
Congo, Dem. Rep.	40	43	47	..	..	..	43	47	51	..	..	..
Congo, Rep.	39	43	47	49	49	25	44	48	53	55	54	21
Costa Rica	60	65	70	74	74	23	63	69	75	78	79	25
Côte d'Ivoire	38	43	49	54	53	40	41	46	52	57	56	37
Croatia	..	..	66	69	70	..	..	..	74	76	78	..
Cuba	62	68	72	73	74	19	66	71	75	77	78	18
Cyprus	67	69	73	74	75	12	71	72	77	79	80	14
Czech Republic	..	..	67	68	70	..	..	..	74	76	77	..
Denmark	70	71	71	72	72	3	74	76	77	78	78	5
Djibouti	35	38	42	46	48	39	38	42	46	50	51	37
Dominica	..	..	..	71	71	..	..	..	..	74	75	..
Dominican Republic	50	57	62	67	68	36	53	60	66	71	72	36
Ecuador	52	56	61	66	67	30	54	59	65	70	72	33
Egypt, Arab Rep.	45	50	54	61	64	41	47	52	57	64	66	39
El Salvador	49	55	52	62	65	33	52	59	63	70	72	39
Equatorial Guinea	35	38	41	45	47	34	38	41	45	49	51	32
Eritrea	38	42	43	47	49	29	41	45	46	50	52	27
Estonia	65	66	64	65	65	0	72	74	74	75	76	5
Ethiopia	34	38	39	45	47	37	38	42	43	48	50	34
Fiji	58	62	66	69	70	22	60	65	70	73	74	23
Finland	65	66	69	71	73	12	72	74	77	79	80	12
France	67	68	70	73	74	10	74	76	78	81	82	11
French Guiana	..	..	..	..	..	..	..	..	..	..	..	..
French Polynesia	..	..	..	65	67	..	..	..	..	70	72	..
Gabon	39	42	46	51	52	34	42	46	50	54	56	33
Gambia, The	31	35	38	42	44	44	34	38	42	46	48	41
Georgia	..	..	67	69	69	..	..	..	75	76	78	..
Germany	67	67	69	72	73	9	72	74	76	78	79	10
Ghana	43	47	51	55	57	30	47	51	54	59	61	30
Greece	67	70	72	75	75	12	70	74	76	80	81	14
Grenada	..	..	..	..	..	..	..	..	..	..	..	..
Guadeloupe	61	64	68	71	72	17	65	70	75	78	79	21
Guam	..	..	..	70	70	..	..	..	..	75	76	..

43

Table 9. Life Expectancy at Birth, 1960–95 (continued)

	Life expectancy at birth (years)											
	Male						Female					
Economy	1960	1970	1980	1990	1995	% change 1960–95	1960	1970	1980	1990	1995	% change 1960–95
Guatemala	45	51	56	61	63	40	46	53	60	66	68	47
Guinea	33	36	39	43	44	34	34	37	40	44	45	31
Guinea-Bissau	34	35	37	41	42	23	35	37	40	44	45	27
Guyana	55	58	58	60	60	11	58	62	64	66	67	16
Haiti	41	46	50	54	54	33	43	49	53	57	57	32
Honduras	45	51	58	63	64	44	48	54	62	68	69	43
Hong Kong, China	61	67	71	75	76	25	69	73	77	80	81	18
Hungary	66	67	66	65	65	–1	70	73	73	74	74	6
Iceland	71	71	74	76	77	8	76	77	80	80	81	7
India	45	50	54	59	62	37	43	48	54	60	63	45
Indonesia	40	47	53	60	62	54	42	49	56	63	66	56
Iran, Islamic Republic	50	55	59	66	68	37	49	54	61	67	69	40
Iraq	48	54	61	61	59	24	49	56	63	63	62	25
Ireland	68	69	70	72	74	8	71	74	75	77	79	11
Israel	70	70	70	74	75	7	73	73	76	78	79	8
Italy	67	69	71	74	74	11	72	75	77	80	81	12
Jamaica	61	66	69	71	72	18	65	69	73	75	76	18
Japan	65	69	73	76	77	17	70	75	79	82	83	18
Jordan	..	..	..	66	68	..	..	..	..	70	72	..
Kazakhstan	..	..	62	64	64	..	..	..	72	73	74	..
Kenya	43	48	53	57	57	33	47	52	57	60	60	29
Kiribati	..	..	..	54	56	..	..	..	..	59	61	..
Korea, Dem. Rep.	52	58	64	66	65	24	56	62	70	73	72	30
Korea, Republic	52	58	64	67	68	30	56	62	70	74	75	36
Kuwait	58	64	69	73	74	27	61	68	73	77	79	29
Kyrgyz Republic	..	..	61	63	63	..	..	..	70	71	72	..
Lao PDR	39	39	43	48	51	30	42	42	46	51	54	29
Latvia	66	66	64	64	63	–4	73	74	74	75	75	3
Lebanon	58	62	63	66	67	16	61	66	67	70	71	16
Lesotho	41	46	51	56	57	40	46	51	55	58	59	31
Liberia	40	45	49	45	45	13	43	48	52	48	46	6
Libya	46	50	55	60	63	38	48	53	59	64	66	38
Lithuania	66	67	66	67	63	–3	72	75	76	76	75	4
Luxembourg	66	67	69	72	73	10	72	74	76	79	80	11
Macao	53	58	64	71	75	41	56	62	69	76	80	41
Macedonia, FYR	..	..	..	70	71	..	..	..	..	73	75	..
Madagascar	39	44	49	54	56	42	42	47	52	57	59	39
Malawi	37	40	43	44	43	16	38	41	45	45	44	15
Malaysia	52	60	65	68	69	32	56	63	69	72	74	33
Maldives	45	51	57	62	64	43	42	49	55	60	62	48
Mali	35	36	41	46	48	36	36	39	43	49	51	41
Malta	67	68	71	73	75	12	70	72	75	78	79	12
Marshall Islands	..	..	..	..	..	..	..	..	..	..	..	..
Martinique	61	65	70	72	73	21	64	71	77	79	80	24
Mauritania	37	41	45	49	51	38	40	44	48	52	54	35
Mauritius	57	60	63	66	68	18	61	64	69	73	74	22
Mayotte	..	..	..	..	..	..	..	..	..	..	..	..
Mexico	55	59	63	67	68	23	59	64	70	73	75	27
Micronesia, Fed. Sts.	..	..	..	61	63	..	..	..	..	64	66	..
Moldova	..	..	62	65	65	..	..	..	69	72	73	..
Mongolia	46	51	56	61	63	39	48	54	59	64	66	38
Montserrat	..	..	..	69	70	..	..	..	..	73	76	..
Morocco	46	50	56	62	64	40	48	53	59	65	67	41
Mozambique	36	40	42	44	45	26	39	43	46	48	48	24
Myanmar	42	47	50	55	57	35	45	50	54	58	61	34
Namibia	41	46	51	55	55	32	44	49	54	57	57	30
Nepal	39	43	48	54	56	45	38	42	47	53	56	47
Netherlands	72	71	72	74	75	4	75	77	79	80	81	7
Netherlands Antilles	..	61	69	74	75	..	..	67	74	79	80	..
New Caledonia	..	..	64	69	71	..	..	..	66	72	75	..
New Zealand	68	69	70	72	73	7	74	75	76	78	79	8
Nicaragua	46	52	56	61	65	41	48	55	61	67	70	44
Niger	34	37	40	43	44	31	37	40	43	47	49	33
Nigeria	38	41	44	48	51	34	41	44	47	51	54	31
Norway	71	71	72	73	75	5	76	77	79	80	81	7
Oman	39	46	58	67	68	74	41	48	60	71	73	77
Pakistan	44	49	54	59	62	39	43	49	55	61	64	49
Panama	60	64	68	70	71	20	62	67	72	75	76	23
Papua New Guinea	41	47	50	54	56	37	40	46	51	56	58	43
Paraguay	62	63	65	66	67	8	66	68	69	70	71	8
Peru	46	52	57	63	65	39	49	55	61	66	68	39
Philippines	51	56	59	62	64	24	54	59	63	66	68	24
Poland	65	67	67	67	67	4	70	74	75	75	76	10
Portugal	61	64	68	70	72	18	66	71	75	77	79	19
Puerto Rico	67	69	70	71	72	8	72	75	77	79	80	12

Table 9. Life Expectancy at Birth, 1960–95 (*continued*)

	Life expectancy at birth (years)											
	Male						Female					
Economy	1960	1970	1980	1990	1995	% change 1960–95	1960	1970	1980	1990	1995	% change 1960–95
Qatar	52	59	64	68	69	35	55	63	69	74	75	37
Reunion	53	59	65	69	70	32	60	66	73	77	79	32
Romania	64	67	67	67	66	4	67	71	72	73	74	9
Russian Federation	..	..	62	64	58	..	..	..	73	74	72	..
Rwanda	41	43	44	39	37	–8	44	46	47	42	40	–10
Samoa	..	..	62	65	67	..	..	..	64	68	71	..
São Tomé and Principe	..	..	..	64	66	..	..	..	..	69	72	..
Saudi Arabia	43	51	60	67	69	58	46	53	62	70	71	56
Senegal	39	42	44	47	49	27	40	43	46	49	51	27
Seychelles	..	..	..	67	68	..	..	..	..	74	76	..
Sierra Leone	30	33	34	34	34	14	33	36	37	37	38	14
Singapore	62	65	69	72	74	21	66	70	74	77	79	20
Slovak Republic	..	..	67	67	68	..	..	..	74	75	76	..
Slovenia	66	66	66	69	70	7	71	73	75	77	78	9
Solomon Islands	..	..	..	61	62	..	..	..	..	62	63	..
Somalia	34	38	41	44	46	35	37	42	44	48	50	32
South Africa	47	50	54	59	61	29	51	56	60	65	67	32
Spain	67	70	73	73	74	10	71	75	79	80	81	14
Sri Lanka	62	64	66	69	70	13	62	66	70	74	75	21
St. Kitts and Nevis	..	..	..	65	67	..	..	..	..	69	71	..
St. Lucia	55	61	..	68	68	24	59	64	..	72	73	25
St. Vincent and the Grenadines	59	62	..	68	69	18	60	64	..	73	76	27
Sudan	38	41	47	50	52	37	41	44	49	52	54	34
Suriname	58	62	63	65	66	14	62	66	67	70	73	18
Swaziland	38	44	49	54	56	47	42	48	54	59	61	46
Sweden	71	72	73	75	76	6	75	77	79	80	81	8
Switzerland	69	70	73	74	75	10	74	76	79	81	82	10
Syrian Arab Republic	49	54	60	64	66	36	51	57	63	68	70	38
Taiwan, China	62	66	70	72	73	18	67	71	75	77	78	15
Tajikistan	56	60	64	67	66	17	61	65	69	72	67	9
Tanzania	39	44	48	50	50	28	42	47	52	53	53	25
Thailand	50	56	61	66	66	32	55	60	65	71	72	32
Togo	38	43	48	50	49	30	41	46	51	53	52	27
Tonga	..	..	..	65	67	..	..	..	..	69	71	..
Trinidad and Tobago	62	63	65	69	70	13	65	68	70	73	75	14
Tunisia	48	53	61	66	68	41	49	54	62	68	70	43
Turkey	49	55	59	64	66	36	52	58	64	68	71	37
Turkmenistan	53	56	61	63	..	..	60	63	68	70	..	..
Turks and Caicos Islands	..	..	..	..	..	..	..	..	..	..	..	..
Uganda	42	49	48	47	44	5	45	50	50	47	44	–3
Ukraine	66	66	65	66	64	–4	72	74	74	75	74	2
United Arab Emirates	52	59	66	72	73	42	55	63	70	75	76	39
United Kingdom	68	69	71	73	74	9	74	75	77	79	79	8
United States	67	67	70	72	74	11	73	75	78	79	80	10
Uruguay	65	66	67	69	70	8	71	72	74	76	77	8
Uzbekistan	..	..	64	66	..	..	..	..	71	72	..	..
Vanuatu	..	..	..	60	62	..	..	..	..	62	65	..
Venezuela	58	62	65	68	69	20	61	68	71	74	75	23
Vietnam	43	53	61	64	65	52	46	56	65	69	70	52
Virgin Islands (UK)	..	..	..	..	..	..	..	..	..	..	..	..
Virgin Islands (US)	..	..	..	71	72	..	..	..	..	77	79	..
West Bank and Gaza	..	..	..	..	..	..	..	..	..	..	..	..
Yemen, Rep.	36	41	47	52	53	47	37	42	50	53	54	47
Yugoslavia, Fed. Republic	62	66	68	69	70	13	64	70	73	74	75	17
Zambia	40	45	49	48	46	14	43	48	52	50	47	8
Zimbabwe	44	49	53	59	56	29	47	52	57	63	59	26
World	49	57	59	63	65	33	51	60	64	68	69	35
Low-income	39	53	57	59	62	59	40	54	59	62	64	60
Excluding China and India	41	45	50	52	55	34	42	47	52	54	57	36
Middle-income	53	57	61	64	65	23	56	61	67	70	71	27
Low- and middle-income	44	55	56	62	63	43	45	56	59	63	66	47
East Asia and Pacific	38	58	63	66	66	74	40	60	66	69	70	75
Europe and Central Asia	62	65	64	65	64	3	67	71	72	73	73	9
Latin America and the Caribbean	54	58	62	65	66	22	58	63	68	71	72	24
Middle East and North Africa	46	52	57	63	65	41	48	53	60	65	68	42
South Asia	44	49	54	59	61	39	43	48	54	59	62	44
Sub-Saharan Africa	39	42	46	49	50	28	42	46	49	52	53	26
High-income	67	68	70	72	74	10	72	74	77	79	81	13

Table 10. Adult Mortality, 1960–95

	Probability of dying between ages 15 and 60 (times 1,000)										
	Male					Female					Both
Economy	1960	1970	1980	1990	1995	1960	1970	1980	1990	1995	1995
Afghanistan	617	556	501	480	455	625	499	435	404	384	420
Albania	201	190	140	127	122	180	113	82	70	65	94
Algeria	343	258	226	193	177	259	201	197	156	133	155
Angola	567	563	569	514	493	503	504	458	420	406	450
Anguilla	..	..	..	..	..	..	..	..	..	..	..
Antigua and Barbuda	..	..	..	142	137	..	..	..	85	72	104
Argentina	217	212	205	188	176	136	116	102	90	84	130
Armenia	228	187	158	216	209	127	99	85	119	108	158
Aruba	..	..	..	..	..	..	..	..	..	..	..
Australia	202	205	167	125	110	118	110	85	68	60	85
Austria	215	209	197	155	148	116	109	92	72	64	106
Azerbaijan	304	247	262	216	231	165	117	127	96	91	161
Bahamas, The	274	274	254	186	174	202	164	118	70	64	119
Bahrain	226	263	215	201	170	163	206	175	147	109	139
Bangladesh	551	473	383	322	314	538	486	388	308	292	303
Barbados	187	193	167	140	128	130	121	98	82	74	101
Belarus	254	196	255	254	301	104	85	95	98	100	200
Belgium	197	193	173	141	135	104	105	90	75	68	101
Belize	..	..	..	194	194	..	..	..	123	100	147
Benin	561	478	486	447	472	465	384	397	369	399	436
Bermuda	..	..	..	..	..	..	..	..	..	..	..
Bhutan	..	..	..	..	..	..	..	..	..	..	..
Bolivia	483	421	357	307	292	355	306	273	250	237	264
Bosnia and Herzegovina	192	182	181	186	..	145	130	108	109	..	..
Botswana	537	472	341	218	212	448	395	278	158	153	183
Brazil	295	248	221	193	181	222	186	161	135	123	152
Brunei	239	173	187	149	140	234	142	132	98	86	113
Bulgaria	174	172	190	211	213	126	106	106	107	106	159
Burkina Faso	586	526	467	429	426	456	407	362	338	340	383
Burundi	568	532	489	460	481	457	432	400	379	403	442
Cambodia	551	509	473	392	370	451	406	355	319	298	334
Cameroon	602	544	489	430	413	486	452	415	361	341	377
Canada	191	188	161	133	125	110	100	85	70	65	95
Cape Verde	384	335	292	245	234	315	279	249	218	206	220
Cayman Islands	..	..	..	..	..	..	..	..	..	..	..
Central African Republic	519	571	540	485	505	442	440	424	381	406	456
Chad	554	554	556	487	470	533	492	449	397	385	428
Channel Islands	..	..	..	133	127	..	..	..	61	52	89
Chile	330	301	218	165	155	240	177	120	92	82	119
China	691	249	185	160	155	631	180	148	135	130	143
Colombia	298	262	237	222	214	237	209	162	127	118	166
Comoros	..	..	..	365	354	..	..	..	307	286	320
Congo, Dem. Rep.	..	..	..	..	..	..	..	..	..	..	..
Congo, Rep.	583	514	408	370	405	448	395	298	273	313	359
Costa Rica	246	180	159	122	115	155	130	100	73	68	92
Côte d'Ivoire	594	526	421	352	392	476	428	346	294	333	363
Croatia	..	..	233	207	176	..	..	106	96	78	127
Cuba	297	163	135	125	122	234	117	94	83	78	100
Cyprus	205	161	131	118	113	150	119	85	72	63	88
Czech Republic	203	221	225	230	195	115	112	102	99	83	139
Denmark	154	156	163	155	145	106	102	102	96	92	119
Djibouti	534	586	527	472	452	519	470	428	387	373	412
Dominica	..	..	..	154	144	..	..	..	113	98	121
Dominican Republic	342	246	183	157	155	271	192	138	109	100	128
Ecuador	312	258	229	183	179	248	208	176	120	110	145
Egypt, Arab Rep.	337	255	257	289	278	246	179	204	248	238	258
El Salvador	363	259	410	284	229	287	193	178	165	154	192
Equatorial Guinea	499	580	543	488	474	491	462	440	400	392	433
Eritrea	..	..	..	433	429	..	..	..	347	342	385
Estonia	238	251	291	286	284	108	104	110	106	95	189
Ethiopia	475	482	491	448	442	391	411	401	358	352	397
Fiji	318	257	209	173	162	264	207	152	115	105	133
Finland	250	263	206	183	150	119	100	74	70	64	107
France	215	202	190	164	155	103	98	85	68	58	107
French Guiana	..	..	..	..	..	..	..	..	..	..	..
French Polynesia	..	..	..	256	232	..	..	..	169	139	185
Gabon	532	521	474	402	386	415	421	387	332	322	354
Gambia, The	578	655	584	530	511	514	519	466	432	419	465
Georgia	283	240	210	195	189	147	113	94	90	77	133
Germany	195	195	177	145	145	114	109	90	73	70	108
Ghana	514	459	400	334	320	419	377	334	270	253	287
Greece	180	145	134	117	113	132	100	86	67	61	87
Grenada	..	..	..	..	..	..	..	..	..	..	..
Guadeloupe	280	223	208	167	153	211	133	99	80	70	112
Guam	..	..	..	183	180	..	..	..	109	97	139

46

Table 10. Adult Mortality, 1960–95 (*continued*)

| Economy | Probability of dying between ages 15 and 60 (times 1,000) | | | | | | | | | | Both |
| | Male | | | | | Female | | | | | |
	1960	1970	1980	1990	1995	1960	1970	1980	1990	1995	1995
Guatemala	514	405	336	264	245	451	342	266	191	166	206
Guinea	526	636	589	529	498	535	534	507	495	497	498
Guinea-Bissau	497	528	535	544	584	530	513	517	533	572	578
Guyana	307	274	294	263	245	249	217	210	172	154	200
Haiti	455	411	348	353	391	347	326	275	291	329	360
Honduras	392	361	306	202	166	290	283	237	141	111	138
Hong Kong, China	301	212	150	122	109	148	112	87	64	57	83
Hungary	190	188	270	290	330	125	116	130	135	138	234
Iceland	163	158	130	109	102	96	86	66	63	59	80
India	398	324	261	236	229	407	353	279	241	219	224
Indonesia	605	478	368	275	262	525	405	308	219	205	233
Iran, Islamic Republic	239	204	221	170	158	220	219	190	174	149	154
Iraq	391	316	207	193	182	324	277	191	154	143	162
Ireland	180	176	175	134	125	135	116	103	78	72	99
Israel	146	155	138	121	105	120	110	85	72	65	85
Italy	185	171	163	130	125	108	92	80	61	57	91
Jamaica	251	199	186	155	144	196	142	121	97	90	117
Japan	215	172	129	108	101	148	104	70	53	47	74
Jordan	..	..	..	205	171	..	..	..	152	120	145
Kazakhstan	371	318	312	306	296	174	149	140	136	120	208
Kenya	547	467	417	357	362	442	379	339	287	295	329
Kiribati	..	..	..	..	..	..	..	..	..	..	..
Korea, Dem. Rep.	391	353	270	223	215	328	278	156	116	102	159
Korea, Rep.	406	356	270	239	230	341	280	156	117	96	163
Kuwait	253	220	172	130	126	202	163	116	80	68	97
Kyrgyz Republic	347	306	296	291	276	193	159	131	143	120	198
Lao PDR	586	610	531	464	444	481	510	439	389	375	410
Latvia	218	248	281	295	328	102	101	106	108	102	215
Lebanon	311	259	241	210	191	250	198	181	150	135	163
Lesotho	450	365	371	384	347	354	277	279	276	258	302
Liberia	479	340	268	254	252	363	241	185	198	198	225
Libya	379	350	276	234	215	292	278	218	185	166	190
Lithuania	154	214	243	246	304	87	94	92	92	97	201
Luxembourg	210	236	195	165	141	117	95	92	85	76	108
Macao	..	..	..	196	..	..	..	..	109	..	..
Macedonia, FYR	..	..	..	147	144	..	..	..	100	92	118
Madagascar	377	351	353	434	445	264	250	278	377	384	415
Malawi	522	479	429	479	553	431	388	349	436	487	520
Malaysia	438	282	230	198	182	369	230	149	125	110	146
Maldives	413	322	247	208	207	449	378	322	284	262	235
Mali	589	537	454	434	412	490	416	362	351	326	369
Malta	192	185	162	134	118	135	126	101	81	72	95
Marshall Islands	..	..	..	..	..	..	..	..	..	..	..
Martinique	291	214	173	141	134	229	132	85	70	66	100
Mauritania	587	539	505	441	467	466	433	416	365	396	432
Mauritius	316	268	277	241	222	255	205	181	126	116	169
Mayotte	..	..	..	..	..	..	..	..	..	..	..
Mexico	306	246	205	173	162	250	188	121	96	89	125
Micronesia, Fed. Sts.	..	..	..	316	295	..	..	..	256	236	265
Moldova	345	321	289	269	275	201	178	173	146	128	202
Mongolia	476	391	320	251	221	396	331	273	211	182	201
Montserrat	..	..	..	167	158	..	..	..	105	86	122
Morocco	370	330	264	234	213	281	258	207	184	163	188
Mozambique	592	498	468	418	431	467	382	361	321	339	385
Myanmar	475	419	384	326	308	372	336	313	267	252	280
Namibia	548	482	427	373	356	454	405	366	318	304	330
Nepal	527	482	376	350	327	507	476	395	376	354	340
Netherlands	144	160	133	118	110	89	86	74	70	65	88
Netherlands Antilles	..	..	..	126	115	..	..	..	71	62	88
New Caledonia	..	..	..	188	149	..	..	..	141	101	125
New Zealand	196	197	177	147	137	112	105	91	77	70	104
Nicaragua	431	348	277	220	177	347	283	189	147	130	153
Niger	543	611	562	515	510	531	490	453	413	401	455
Nigeria	551	605	535	476	450	429	502	453	401	377	414
Norway	160	164	144	125	118	85	78	71	66	60	89
Oman	423	466	389	217	201	325	390	326	157	134	167
Pakistan	420	339	283	232	208	456	381	291	247	228	218
Panama	273	225	172	146	139	241	185	117	94	88	113
Papua New Guinea	521	496	514	425	371	495	483	478	386	339	355
Paraguay	219	211	198	169	158	166	157	144	117	108	133
Peru	404	348	287	228	211	324	282	229	173	157	184
Philippines	449	376	323	273	254	379	314	259	208	189	222
Poland	177	204	253	263	179	115	104	105	102	92	136
Portugal	198	184	199	177	163	131	100	95	83	76	120
Puerto Rico	167	169	159	158	147	110	89	78	67	61	104

47

Table 10. Adult Mortality, 1960–95 (continued)

Economy	Male 1960	1970	1980	1990	1995	Female 1960	1970	1980	1990	1995	Both 1995
Qatar	243	275	224	194	177	175	219	159	112	100	139
Reunion	316	309	282	213	187	208	180	121	85	74	131
Romania	195	186	216	237	270	140	120	116	114	119	195
Russian Federation	228	278	341	298	472	100	102	120	107	172	322
Rwanda	545	502	503	493	542	438	403	409	409	461	502
Samoa	..	..	..	262	222	..	..	..	202	158	190
São Tomé and Principe	..	..	..	153	149	..	..	..	104	84	117
Saudi Arabia	419	345	283	192	181	326	275	241	158	149	165
Senegal	570	572	586	579	561	477	489	516	506	496	529
Seychelles	367	328	299	221	203	294	268	237	113	90	147
Sierra Leone	585	552	540	601	589	522	534	527	492	470	529
Singapore	305	232	199	138	130	210	138	115	80	75	103
Slovak Republic	..	..	226	247	221	..	..	105	100	93	157
Slovenia	213	238	250	211	188	123	116	105	91	81	134
Solomon Islands	..	..	..	299	300	..	..	..	273	268	284
Somalia	687	592	500	426	399	599	476	412	337	313	356
South Africa	568	516	..	..	..	457	420	..	..	..	..
Spain	177	169	144	146	140	113	95	69	62	57	99
Sri Lanka	204	214	210	184	172	238	196	152	120	108	140
St. Kitts and Nevis	..	..	..	227	204	..	..	..	165	133	169
St. Lucia	..	..	..	205	200	..	..	..	144	126	163
St. Vincent and the Grenadines	..	..	..	202	187	..	..	..	119	93	140
Sudan	611	615	537	464	445	499	525	462	398	378	411
Suriname	294	253	250	216	205	235	191	187	137	106	155
Swaziland	604	447	321	260	248	486	336	232	196	191	220
Sweden	141	141	142	119	102	95	84	76	65	60	81
Switzerland	173	162	145	128	115	99	91	70	64	58	87
Syrian Arab Republic	..	..	..	237	217	..	..	..	177	154	186
Taiwan, China	264	209	190	176	160	181	136	..	91	82	121
Tajikistan	253	217	190	168	200	182	153	129	106	197	199
Tanzania	606	513	451	444	485	498	419	370	373	417	451
Thailand	395	327	280	207	199	313	259	210	123	119	159
Togo	548	529	457	389	377	427	431	375	321	311	344
Tonga	..	..	..	260	231	..	..	..	194	156	193
Trinidad and Tobago	270	231	234	180	170	225	181	166	160	130	150
Tunisia	324	276	227	190	171	270	249	224	174	148	160
Turkey	182	155	153	165	158	108	99	98	118	111	135
Turkmenistan	326	289	263	250	250	205	177	154	135	122	186
Turks and Caicos Islands	..	..	..	..	..	..	..	..	..	..	..
Uganda	549	447	463	526	622	451	393	395	461	558	590
Ukraine	190	239	282	268	294	103	105	112	105	112	203
United Arab Emirates	243	229	153	130	122	175	179	106	101	92	107
United Kingdom	183	175	160	130	120	106	103	96	75	69	95
United States	231	237	194	175	160	130	128	102	90	85	123
Uruguay	187	183	176	178	174	105	98	91	90	83	129
Uzbekistan	289	254	219	207	209	181	147	116	109	101	155
Vanuatu	..	..	..	288	275	..	..	..	241	219	247
Venezuela	276	231	219	186	173	224	157	123	101	94	133
Vietnam	460	320	262	215	206	356	256	204	153	136	171
Virgin Islands (UK)	..	..	..	..	..	..	..	..	..	..	..
Virgin Islands (US)	..	..	..	148	133	..	..	..	78	63	98
West Bank and Gaza	..	..	..	..	..	..	..	..	..	..	..
Yemen, Rep.	539	449	382	363	384	469	388	304	336	331	358
Yugoslavia, Fed. Republic	172	166	164	168	170	148	121	106	101	99	134
Zambia	607	546	482	434	534	506	460	413	377	494	514
Zimbabwe	571	469	389	305	391	482	391	321	270	393	392
World	420	285	250	230	220	340	230	200	175	160	190
Low-income	580	335	280	255	240	470	295	240	220	210	225
Excluding China and India	485	435	385	360	350	400	360	320	310	300	325
Middle-income	310	275	255	220	240	270	230	205	180	150	195
Low- and middle-income	500	320	270	250	240	410	260	235	215	190	215
East Asia and Pacific	660	285	230	215	200	540	230	180	160	150	175
Europe and Central Asia	180	165	180	210	290	150	135	135	125	120	205
Latin America and the Caribbean	295	245	210	195	180	240	200	170	140	110	145
Middle East and North Africa	310	270	240	220	210	255	210	195	185	180	195
South Asia	465	390	315	275	240	400	360	280	250	230	235
Sub-Saharan Africa	520	490	440	400	430	420	405	360	330	360	395
High-income	180	170	140	135	130	150	140	110	80	60	95

Table 11. Total Fertility Rate, 1960–95

Economy	Total fertility rate					Percentage change	
	1960	1970	1980	1990	1995	1960–95	1980–95
Afghanistan	6.9	7.1	7.1	6.9	6.9	−1	−2
Albania	6.9	5.2	3.6	3.0	2.6	−61	−27
Algeria	7.3	7.4	6.8	4.6	3.6	−51	−47
Angola	6.4	6.5	6.9	7.2	6.9	9	1
Anguilla	..	..	..	..	..	..	..
Antigua and Barbuda	..	..	2.2	1.8	1.7	..	−21
Argentina	3.1	3.1	3.3	2.9	2.7	−12	−17
Armenia	4.5	3.2	2.3	2.8	1.8	−60	−22
Aruba	..	..	..	..	..	..	..
Australia	3.5	2.9	1.9	1.9	1.9	−45	−2
Austria	2.7	2.3	1.6	1.5	1.5	−46	−10
Azerbaijan	5.5	4.7	3.2	2.7	2.3	−59	−29
Bahamas, The	3.7	3.5	3.3	2.1	2.0	−47	−41
Bahrain	7.1	6.6	5.3	3.8	3.2	−55	−39
Bangladesh	7.1	7.0	6.2	4.4	3.5	−50	−43
Barbados	4.5	3.1	2.1	1.8	1.8	−60	−12
Belarus	2.7	2.4	2.0	1.9	1.4	−49	−31
Belgium	2.6	2.2	1.7	1.6	1.6	−37	−3
Belize	..	6.9	..	4.4	3.9	..	..
Benin	6.8	6.9	6.5	6.4	6.1	−11	−7
Bermuda	..	..	..	..	..	..	..
Bhutan	..	..	..	..	..	..	..
Bolivia	6.7	6.5	5.6	4.9	4.6	−32	−17
Bosnia and Herzegovina	4.0	2.9	2.1	1.7	..	..	..
Botswana	6.8	6.9	6.7	5.0	4.4	−35	−34
Brazil	6.2	5.0	4.0	2.8	2.4	−60	−38
Brunei	6.9	5.7	4.1	3.3	3.0	−57	−28
Bulgaria	2.3	2.2	2.1	1.7	1.2	−46	−40
Burkina Faso	6.7	7.0	7.5	7.1	6.8	1	−10
Burundi	6.8	6.8	6.8	6.8	6.5	−4	−4
Cambodia	6.3	5.9	4.6	4.9	4.7	−25	3
Cameroon	4.9	5.7	6.5	5.8	5.7	17	−12
Canada	3.8	2.3	1.7	1.8	1.7	−56	−3
Cape Verde	7.0	7.0	6.5	4.5	4.0	−42	−38
Cayman Islands	..	..	..	..	..	..	..
Central African Republic	5.6	5.7	5.8	5.5	5.1	−9	−11
Chad	6.0	6.0	5.9	5.9	5.9	−1	0
Channel Islands	..	..	1.4	1.7	1.7	..	18
Chile	5.3	4.0	2.9	2.6	2.4	−56	−18
China	3.4	5.8	2.5	2.1	1.9	−43	−24
Colombia	6.8	5.5	3.8	3.1	2.8	−59	−27
Comoros	..	..	..	6.3	6.0	..	..
Congo, Dem. Rep.	6.0	6.2	6.6	..	..	..	..
Congo, Rep.	5.4	5.9	6.1	6.3	6.1	13	−1
Costa Rica	7.0	5.1	3.7	3.3	2.9	−59	−22
Côte d'Ivoire	7.2	7.4	7.4	6.3	5.4	−26	−28
Croatia	..	..	..	1.6	1.5	..	..
Cuba	4.2	3.9	2.0	1.8	1.7	−59	−16
Cyprus	3.5	2.6	2.5	2.4	2.2	−37	−11
Czech Republic	2.1	1.9	2.1	1.9	1.3	−38	−38
Denmark	2.6	2.0	1.5	1.7	1.8	−30	16
Djibouti	6.6	6.6	6.6	6.0	5.8	−12	−12
Dominica	..	..	..	2.8	2.4	..	..
Dominican Republic	7.4	6.2	4.3	3.3	2.9	−60	−31
Ecuador	6.9	6.4	5.0	3.7	3.3	−53	−35
Egypt, Arab Rep.	7.0	6.1	5.2	4.0	3.5	−50	−32
El Salvador	6.8	6.4	5.4	4.0	3.7	−46	−31
Equatorial Guinea	5.5	5.7	5.7	5.9	5.9	7	3
Eritrea	..	..	..	5.8	5.8	..	..
Estonia	2.0	2.2	2.0	2.0	1.3	−33	−35
Ethiopia	5.8	5.8	6.5	7.0	7.0	21	8
Fiji	6.4	4.2	3.6	3.1	2.8	−56	−22
Finland	2.7	1.8	1.6	1.8	1.8	−33	11
France	2.7	2.5	1.9	1.8	1.7	−38	−13
French Guiana	..	..	..	..	..	..	..
French Polynesia	..	5.6	..	3.4	3.0	..	..
Gabon	4.1	4.2	4.4	5.0	5.2	28	17
Gambia, The	6.4	6.5	6.5	5.9	5.3	−17	−18
Georgia	..	2.7	2.3	2.2	..	..	..
Germany	2.4	2.0	1.6	1.5	1.2	−48	−21
Ghana	6.9	6.7	6.5	5.9	5.2	−25	−20
Greece	2.3	2.3	2.2	1.4	1.4	−41	−39
Grenada	..	..	..	..	..	..	..
Guadeloupe	5.6	4.9	2.8	2.3	2.1	−62	−25
Guam	6.0	4.7	..	2.9	2.7	−55	..

Table 11. Total Fertility Rate, 1960–95 (*continued*)

Economy	Total fertility rate					Percentage change	
	1960	*1970*	*1980*	*1990*	*1995*	*1960–95*	*1980–95*
Guatemala	6.9	6.5	6.3	5.4	4.8	−30	−23
Guinea	5.9	6.0	6.1	6.5	6.5	11	7
Guinea-Bissau	5.9	5.9	6.0	6.0	6.0	3	0
Guyana	6.5	5.5	3.6	2.6	2.4	−62	−32
Haiti	6.3	6.0	5.9	5.2	4.5	−29	−24
Honduras	7.3	7.4	6.5	5.1	4.7	−36	−28
Hong Kong, China	5.0	3.5	2.1	1.3	1.2	−75	−40
Hungary	2.0	2.0	1.9	1.8	1.6	−22	−18
Iceland	4.3	2.8	2.5	2.3	2.1	−50	−14
India	6.6	5.8	5.0	3.8	3.2	−51	−35
Indonesia	5.4	5.5	4.4	3.1	2.7	−50	−39
Iran, Islamic Republic	7.2	6.8	6.1	5.6	4.6	−37	−26
Iraq	7.2	7.1	6.5	5.9	5.5	−24	−15
Ireland	3.8	3.9	3.2	2.1	1.9	−50	−42
Israel	3.9	3.8	3.3	2.8	2.4	−38	−26
Italy	2.4	2.4	1.6	1.3	1.2	−51	−29
Jamaica	5.4	5.4	3.8	2.9	2.5	−54	−35
Japan	2.0	2.1	1.8	1.5	1.5	−25	−14
Jordan	..	..	6.9	5.4	4.8	..	−30
Kazakhstan	..	3.4	2.9	2.7	2.3	..	−22
Kenya	8.0	8.1	7.9	5.8	4.8	−40	−39
Kiribati	..	..	4.6	4.1	3.8	..	−17
Korea, Dem. Rep.	5.8	6.4	3.1	2.4	2.2	−61	−28
Korea, Rep.	5.7	4.3	2.6	1.8	1.8	−69	−33
Kuwait	7.3	7.2	5.4	3.5	3.0	−59	−44
Kyrgyz Republic	..	4.9	4.1	3.7	3.3	..	−20
Lao PDR	6.2	6.2	6.7	6.7	6.5	6	−2
Latvia	1.9	1.9	2.0	2.0	1.3	−34	−38
Lebanon	6.3	5.5	4.0	3.3	2.9	−54	−29
Lesotho	5.8	5.7	5.6	5.1	4.7	−20	−17
Liberia	6.6	6.8	6.8	6.8	6.6	−1	−3
Libya	7.1	7.5	7.3	6.2	4.1	−42	−44
Lithuania	2.5	2.4	2.0	2.0	1.5	−41	−24
Luxembourg	2.3	2.0	1.5	1.6	1.7	−26	12
Macao	5.6	4.6	..	2.3	1.9	−67	..
Macedonia, FYR	..	3.1	2.5	2.2	2.2	..	−14
Madagascar	6.6	6.6	6.5	6.3	5.9	−11	−10
Malawi	7.8	7.8	7.6	7.2	6.6	−15	−13
Malaysia	6.8	5.5	4.2	3.8	3.4	−50	−19
Maldives	7.0	7.0	6.9	6.8	6.7	−5	−4
Mali	7.1	7.1	7.1	7.1	6.9	−4	−4
Malta	3.6	2.0	2.0	2.1	1.9	−48	−8
Marshall Islands	..	..	..	..	..	..	..
Martinique	5.6	4.5	2.4	2.1	2.0	−64	−15
Mauritania	6.5	6.5	6.3	5.6	5.2	−20	−17
Mauritius	5.9	3.8	2.8	2.2	2.2	−62	−20
Mayotte	..	..	..	..	..	..	..
Mexico	6.8	6.5	4.6	3.5	3.0	−55	−34
Micronesia, Fed. Sts.	..	..	..	4.9	4.6	..	..
Moldova	..	2.6	2.4	2.4	2.0	..	−18
Mongolia	6.0	5.9	5.4	4.2	3.4	−43	−37
Montserrat	..	..	..	2.5	2.3	..	..
Morocco	7.2	7.0	5.5	4.1	3.5	−52	−37
Mozambique	6.3	6.5	6.5	6.5	6.3	−1	−3
Myanmar	6.0	5.9	5.1	3.9	3.5	−43	−32
Namibia	6.0	6.0	5.9	5.4	5.0	−16	−15
Nepal	5.8	6.3	6.4	5.7	5.3	−8	−17
Netherlands	3.1	2.6	1.6	1.6	1.6	−49	−1
Netherlands Antilles	5.1	3.0	2.4	2.1	2.1	−59	−11
New Caledonia	..	4.3	3.8	2.9	2.5	..	−34
New Zealand	4.0	3.2	2.1	2.2	2.1	−48	−1
Nicaragua	7.4	7.0	6.2	4.7	4.2	−43	−32
Niger	7.1	7.2	7.4	7.4	7.4	4	0
Nigeria	6.8	6.9	6.9	6.0	5.6	−18	−19
Norway	2.8	2.5	1.7	1.9	1.9	−34	9
Oman	7.2	8.2	10.0	7.8	7.1	−2	−29
Pakistan	6.9	7.0	7.0	5.9	5.3	−23	−24
Panama	5.9	5.3	3.8	3.0	2.7	−54	−29
Papua New Guinea	6.3	6.1	5.7	5.2	4.8	−23	−15
Paraguay	6.8	6.0	4.9	4.5	4.1	−40	−16
Peru	6.9	6.1	4.6	3.5	3.2	−54	−31
Philippines	7.0	6.4	4.9	4.1	3.8	−46	−23
Poland	3.0	2.2	2.3	2.1	1.6	−46	−29
Portugal	3.0	2.8	2.2	1.5	1.4	−52	−34
Puerto Rico	4.6	3.2	2.6	2.2	2.1	−54	−17

Table 11. Total Fertility Rate, 1960–95 (*continued*)

Economy	Total fertility rate 1960	1970	1980	1990	1995	Percentage change 1960–95	1980–95
Qatar	7.0	6.9	5.8	4.4	3.9	−44	−32
Reunion	5.8	4.4	3.1	2.4	2.2	−62	−29
Romania	2.3	2.9	2.4	1.8	1.4	−40	−42
Russian Federation	2.6	2.0	1.9	1.9	1.4	−46	−26
Rwanda	7.5	8.1	8.3	6.8	6.3	−17	−24
Samoa	..	6.7	..	4.8	4.3	..	..
São Tomé and Principe	..	..	..	5.1	4.8	..	..
Saudi Arabia	7.2	7.3	7.3	6.6	6.3	−13	−14
Senegal	6.4	6.5	6.7	6.2	5.8	−11	−14
Seychelles	..	..	..	2.8	2.5	..	..
Sierra Leone	6.2	6.4	6.5	6.5	6.5	4	0
Singapore	5.5	3.1	1.7	1.9	1.7	−69	−2
Slovak Republic	3.1	2.4	2.3	2.1	1.5	−50	−34
Slovenia	2.4	2.3	2.1	1.5	1.3	−45	−38
Solomon Islands	..	..	6.8	5.7	5.2	..	−23
Somalia	7.0	7.0	7.0	7.0	7.0	0	0
South Africa	6.5	5.7	4.9	4.2	3.9	−40	−21
Spain	2.9	2.8	2.2	1.3	1.2	−59	−47
Sri Lanka	5.3	4.3	3.5	2.5	2.3	−56	−34
St. Kitts and Nevis	..	..	..	2.7	2.4	..	..
St. Lucia	6.9	..	4.4	3.3	3.0	−57	−32
St. Vincent and the Grenadines	7.3	..	..	2.6	2.3	−68	..
Sudan	6.7	6.7	6.5	5.2	4.8	−28	−27
Suriname	6.6	5.6	4.4	3.2	2.6	−60	−39
Swaziland	6.5	6.5	6.3	5.1	4.7	−28	−26
Sweden	2.2	1.9	1.7	2.1	1.7	−20	4
Switzerland	2.3	2.1	1.6	1.6	1.5	−37	−5
Syrian Arab Republic	7.3	7.7	7.4	5.9	4.9	−33	−34
Taiwan, China	5.7	3.8	2.6	1.9	1.8	−69	−33
Tajikistan	6.3	6.8	5.6	5.1	4.2	−34	−26
Tanzania	6.8	6.8	6.8	6.1	5.8	−15	−14
Thailand	6.4	5.6	3.6	2.3	1.8	−71	−49
Togo	6.6	6.6	6.6	6.6	6.4	−2	−2
Tonga	..	..	4.9	3.9	3.3	..	−32
Trinidad and Tobago	5.2	3.6	3.3	2.5	2.1	−58	−35
Tunisia	7.1	6.5	5.3	3.6	3.0	−58	−43
Turkey	6.3	5.3	4.3	3.3	2.7	−57	−37
Turkmenistan	6.4	6.3	4.9	4.2	3.8	−41	−24
Turks and Caicos Islands	..	..	..	..	..	..	..
Uganda	6.9	7.1	7.2	7.0	6.8	−3	−6
Ukraine	2.2	2.0	2.0	1.8	1.5	−32	−25
United Arab Emirates	6.9	6.6	5.4	4.2	3.6	−48	−33
United Kingdom	2.7	2.4	1.9	1.8	1.7	−36	−10
United States	3.7	2.5	1.8	2.1	2.1	−44	12
Uruguay	2.9	2.9	2.7	2.4	2.2	−22	−18
Uzbekistan	..	5.7	4.8	4.1	3.7	..	−23
Vanuatu	..	..	..	5.6	5.0	..	..
Venezuela	6.5	5.4	4.2	3.5	3.1	−52	−26
Viet Nam	6.1	5.9	5.1	3.6	3.1	−49	−39
Virgin Islands (UK)	..	..	..	..	..	..	..
Virgin Islands (US)	5.6	5.3	..	2.6	2.4	−57	..
West Bank and Gaza	..	..	..	..	..	..	..
Yemen, Rep.	7.5	7.7	7.9	7.6	7.4	−2	−6
Yugoslavia, Fed. Republic	2.7	2.4	2.3	2.1	1.9	−30	−20
Zambia	6.6	6.8	7.1	6.2	5.7	−13	−19
Zimbabwe	8.0	7.8	6.8	4.9	3.9	−51	−43
World	4.9	5.1	3.7	3.1	2.9	−41	−22
Low-income	5.2	5.5	4.3	3.5	3.2	−38	−26
Excluding China and India	6.6	6.4	6.3	5.4	5.0	−24	−21
Middle-income	4.9	4.4	3.8	3.1	3.0	−39	−21
Low- and middle-income	5.1	5.2	4.1	3.8	3.1	−39	−24
East Asia and Pacific	4.1	5.8	3.1	2.4	2.2	−46	−29
Latin America and the Caribbean	6.0	5.3	4.1	3.2	2.8	−53	−32
Middle East and North Africa	7.2	6.8	6.1	5.0	4.2	−42	−31
South Asia	6.6	6.0	5.3	4.1	3.5	−47	−34
Sub-Saharan Africa	6.6	6.6	6.7	6.1	5.7	−14	−15
High-income	3.0	2.5	1.9	1.7	1.7	−43	−11

Table 12. The Aging Population, 1995 and 2020

Economy	Population over age 60 (percentage of total) Male 1995	Male 2020	Female 1995	Female 2020	Probability of surviving to age 60 (percentage of birth cohort) Male 1995	Male 2020	Female 1995	Female 2020
Afghanistan	4.6	4.4	5.1	4.7	40.7	51.9	42.2	55.0
Albania	8.2	13.5	10.3	16.5	81.3	85.6	88.8	92.7
Algeria	5.4	9.1	6.2	10.0	78.3	85.7	82.6	90.6
Angola	4.3	3.9	5.1	4.7	42.6	51.7	48.3	58.6
Anguilla	..	..	..	..	..	..	..	..
Antigua and Barbuda	6.7	7.5	11.4	16.3	83.6	87.6	90.8	94.5
Argentina	11.5	14.1	14.8	18.3	79.6	85.3	89.2	92.7
Armenia	9.7	13.7	12.2	18.5	76.4	82.9	86.5	91.4
Aruba	..	..	..	..	..	..	..	..
Australia	13.6	21.4	16.6	24.7	86.2	89.7	92.9	95.1
Austria	16.0	25.5	23.4	30.3	86.1	90.2	92.8	95.2
Azerbaijan	7.8	11.2	10.8	16.8	75.1	82.7	88.4	93.4
Bahamas, The	7.2	11.7	8.0	15.4	80.6	86.2	89.7	93.7
Bahrain	4.9	..	5.2	12.1	81.8	87.0	87.7	92.0
Bangladesh	5.5	7.7	4.5	7.9	59.8	72.6	62.6	77.1
Barbados	10.9	17.3	16.8	21.4	85.5	89.4	91.5	94.3
Belarus	13.1	18.2	21.3	26.8	68.3	77.4	88.3	93.2
Belgium	18.4	25.3	24.1	30.5	85.2	88.6	92.6	94.8
Belize	6.5	6.9	6.5	8.1	84.7	88.3	88.2	92.9
Benin	4.1	4.0	4.7	4.7	46.6	54.0	52.2	58.9
Bermuda	..	..	..	..	..	..	..	..
Bhutan	4.9	5.0	6.1	7.4	49.6	61.3	55.9	68.3
Bolivia	5.5	6.7	6.4	8.3	62.7	74.0	68.2	79.4
Bosnia and Herzegovina	10.8	19.2	14.0	24.8	79.6	85.1	88.0	93.1
Botswana	2.7	4.2	4.4	5.7	42.3	51.0	49.5	58.2
Brazil	7.0	11.1	7.9	14.1	68.8	76.6	82.6	88.4
Brunei	6.0	15.7	5.9	16.3	84.9	88.8	90.7	94.3
Bulgaria	18.8	22.2	22.6	28.5	76.4	83.0	87.7	91.5
Burkina Faso	4.6	3.0	4.9	3.9	39.6	48.5	43.4	53.2
Burundi	3.2	3.8	4.7	4.8	37.2	50.6	43.6	57.9
Cambodia	3.4	5.0	5.1	7.6	51.6	57.5	56.7	63.8
Cameroon	5.0	4.6	5.8	5.4	54.2	65.2	60.6	72.0
Canada	14.1	24.7	17.7	28.5	87.8	91.0	93.7	95.7
Cape Verde	5.7	3.1	8.4	6.9	71.0	78.1	73.7	82.2
Cayman Islands	..	..	..	..	..	..	..	..
Central African Republic	5.3	5.1	6.6	6.6	41.3	50.3	50.7	59.7
Chad	5.4	5.5	6.3	6.4	45.0	54.1	50.7	61.4
Channel Islands	20.3	27.3	23.3	34.2	86.2	89.5	93.9	96.1
Chile	7.9	14.7	10.8	18.5	82.4	87.3	90.9	94.1
China	9.3	15.2	10.1	16.5	78.2	82.9	82.5	88.1
Colombia	7.4	10.3	8.0	13.6	75.2	82.5	85.3	90.8
Comoros	4.0	4.4	4.4	5.7	55.8	64.6	62.3	77.2
Congo, Dem. Rep.	4.0	3.6	5.0	4.3	49.2	59.4	54.8	65.4
Congo, Rep.	4.7	3.6	6.6	5.2	45.7	53.9	55.3	67.5
Costa Rica	6.5	12.9	7.5	14.8	86.5	89.6	91.7	94.3
Côte d'Ivoire	4.6	5.4	4.4	5.2	54.2	62.5	58.8	67.2
Croatia	16.0	24.8	22.9	31.2	80.2	86.8	90.6	94.1
Cuba	11.8	18.6	12.7	21.8	86.4	89.5	91.1	94.0
Cyprus	12.6	20.0	15.5	24.0	87.6	90.3	92.7	95.5
Czech Republic	14.9	22.5	21.0	28.9	78.7	85.8	90.1	93.7
Denmark	17.1	24.2	21.8	28.7	83.7	87.4	91.1	93.7
Djibouti	4.2	5.0	4.9	5.8	47.2	57.8	52.8	64.5
Dominica	10.8	8.0	10.8	10.0	83.0	87.3	88.3	93.3
Dominican Republic	5.9	11.1	6.3	13.4	78.5	84.9	85.9	92.3
Ecuador	5.8	9.7	6.7	11.5	76.9	84.3	84.5	90.7
Egypt, Arab Rep.	5.8	9.9	7.1	10.9	69.0	80.9	71.3	83.1
El Salvador	5.2	5.9	6.5	8.8	73.1	81.7	84.5	89.8
Equatorial Guinea	6.1	5.1	6.4	6.1	45.4	56.1	51.1	62.9
Eritrea	3.5	4.1	4.1	5.0	43.4	52.9	49.8	61.5
Estonia	14.7	21.1	22.9	31.7	70.3	80.0	88.8	93.8
Ethiopia	3.9	4.4	5.0	4.9	45.9	55.8	51.5	62.2
Fiji	6.1	12.8	6.5	15.1	81.1	86.3	87.1	91.7
Finland	15.0	25.2	22.2	30.5	83.6	88.2	92.7	95.1
France	16.6	24.3	22.4	29.7	85.9	89.9	93.9	95.9
French Guiana	..	..	..	..	..	..	..	..
French Polynesia	6.1	8.9	6.4	10.7	74.7	84.4	84.0	92.3
Gabon	8.1	7.5	9.5	8.6	53.6	60.4	60.1	70.3
Gambia, The	4.5	6.1	4.8	7.0	41.1	51.7	46.9	58.9
Georgia	13.9	18.7	19.8	27.5	79.1	85.2	90.5	94.4
Germany	16.5	27.0	24.1	31.3	85.3	89.3	92.3	94.8
Ghana	4.4	5.7	5.1	6.7	59.9	68.4	66.9	76.8
Greece	19.9	25.0	23.3	29.7	87.5	90.6	93.1	95.4
Grenada	9.1	6.1	10.6	13.7	78.0	85.1	87.8	93.2
Guadeloupe	9.6	15.5	12.4	19.8	83.1	87.6	91.7	95.1
Guam	6.3	14.9	7.0	16.3	80.4	85.6	89.2	93.6

52

Table 12. The Aging Population, 1995 and 2020 (*continued*)

Economy	Population over age 60 (percentage of total)				Probability of surviving to age 60 (percentage of birth cohort)			
	Male		Female		Male		Female	
	1995	2020	1995	2020	1995	2020	1995	2020
Guatemala	4.9	5.3	5.4	6.5	69.3	79.7	77.8	87.5
Guinea	4.0	4.2	4.5	4.1	42.4	51.1	40.9	49.7
Guinea-Bissau	4.4	2.8	5.3	4.1	29.0	38.3	30.7	40.2
Guyana	5.8	9.4	6.7	12.2	65.6	68.8	77.5	79.2
Haiti	5.5	5.8	6.6	7.6	53.1	59.6	59.1	63.5
Honduras	4.5	6.0	5.0	7.2	72.2	80.8	79.3	87.6
Hong Kong, China	13.3	27.9	15.2	29.4	88.1	90.6	93.6	95.5
Hungary	16.1	20.6	22.3	27.7	70.9	79.0	87.0	91.2
Iceland	12.6	20.4	16.5	23.3	88.6	90.9	93.6	95.5
India	7.3	10.6	7.9	11.3	68.9	77.2	70.0	81.3
Indonesia	6.2	10.4	7.0	11.8	68.0	78.4	73.7	84.1
Iran, Islamic Republic	6.0	7.4	5.7	7.9	78.7	85.0	79.5	88.3
Iraq	4.5	6.4	5.0	7.1	67.5	83.7	71.9	89.2
Ireland	13.8	18.5	16.9	22.1	86.6	90.7	92.5	95.5
Israel	10.0	15.4	12.2	17.4	87.3	90.3	91.8	94.5
Italy	19.5	26.8	24.8	32.6	86.6	90.2	93.4	95.6
Jamaica	8.1	11.1	9.6	13.8	83.4	87.9	89.6	93.2
Japan	17.8	28.7	22.3	34.0	89.0	91.3	94.6	96.3
Jordan	4.9	6.6	4.0	7.4	77.8	85.9	82.8	90.9
Kazakhstan	9.1	13.6	13.7	20.2	69.8	78.0	86.8	92.4
Kenya	4.0	4.9	4.5	5.6	58.3	65.5	64.6	70.9
Kiribati	5.0	7.3	5.3	9.3	57.9	73.8	67.4	83.7
Korea, Dem. Rep.	5.1	12.2	8.7	15.5	74.9	82.6	86.5	92.5
Korea, Rep.	7.3	16.4	10.7	21.7	75.3	83.3	89.0	93.6
Kuwait	3.8	13.3	3.4	13.5	85.7	88.7	91.9	94.4
Kyrgyz Republic	7.4	9.2	10.8	13.7	66.4	75.0	82.6	90.6
Lao PDR	4.5	5.0	5.3	5.7	49.4	60.8	54.7	67.3
Latvia	15.2	21.3	23.9	32.6	66.6	76.7	88.0	93.1
Lebanon	7.8	7.7	8.6	11.4	70.1	78.1	77.2	85.4
Lesotho	5.3	6.7	6.7	8.0	60.8	67.5	64.9	72.9
Liberia	4.1	5.3	4.6	4.9	43.6	67.6	44.5	66.2
Libya	4.6	5.9	4.0	5.8	70.0	80.4	77.0	88.5
Lithuania	13.3	18.9	20.6	27.6	68.8	77.1	88.1	92.4
Luxembourg	16.5	25.6	21.6	29.8	84.8	88.8	92.6	95.1
Macao	8.2	22.2	10.0	22.6	87.0	90.0	92.4	95.2
Macedonia, FYR	11.8	20.3	14.7	23.7	83.2	88.1	88.1	93.5
Madagascar	4.4	4.9	5.1	5.8	59.5	69.0	64.5	74.8
Malawi	3.9	4.0	4.5	4.3	40.5	48.6	41.0	48.6
Malaysia	5.4	9.9	6.3	12.1	78.9	85.3	86.7	91.6
Maldives	5.3	5.8	5.0	5.3	72.9	81.9	67.6	83.7
Mali	3.8	4.0	4.7	5.0	47.0	60.0	53.3	66.8
Malta	13.7	22.7	16.9	26.5	86.1	89.6	91.6	94.4
Marshall Islands	..	..	..	..	..	..	..	..
Martinique	11.9	17.0	15.4	22.9	85.4	89.2	92.7	95.6
Mauritania	4.7	5.6	5.8	6.5	50.6	59.9	56.2	67.1
Mauritius	7.5	14.1	9.2	17.2	75.9	82.7	86.9	91.1
Mayotte	..	..	..	..	..	..	..	..
Mexico	5.4	9.7	6.6	12.3	79.1	85.2	87.3	91.9
Micronesia, Fed. Sts.	3.6	5.3	5.8	6.6	66.7	76.7	72.3	83.1
Moldova	11.3	16.1	16.1	23.1	70.3	79.0	83.9	91.7
Mongolia	5.0	8.9	6.0	10.1	71.2	81.7	75.1	86.1
Montserrat	16.7	0.0	16.7	12.5	80.5	86.0	88.6	93.5
Morocco	5.9	9.1	6.5	10.8	71.6	80.8	77.0	86.3
Mozambique	4.5	4.4	5.4	5.2	41.2	50.4	46.7	56.1
Myanmar	6.3	8.4	7.3	9.9	61.6	72.1	67.0	78.0
Namibia	5.1	5.6	6.0	6.7	54.3	63.1	58.3	71.8
Nepal	5.5	6.0	5.3	6.6	60.6	68.5	57.7	68.0
Netherlands	15.8	26.7	20.4	30.4	87.0	90.2	93.3	95.4
Netherlands Antilles	9.2	16.5	11.8	22.2	86.8	90.0	92.5	95.5
New Caledonia	8.5	13.5	8.8	15.1	82.7	88.3	87.8	94.2
New Zealand	13.3	19.2	16.1	22.9	85.2	89.2	92.0	94.6
Nicaragua	4.3	6.7	4.9	7.9	73.3	84.2	81.3	89.7
Niger	3.9	3.3	4.6	4.3	40.5	47.6	49.4	60.3
Nigeria	3.6	5.5	4.5	6.4	52.7	66.5	58.6	72.6
Norway	17.7	24.3	22.7	27.7	87.0	90.5	93.3	95.4
Oman	3.6	6.5	4.4	5.0	77.5	84.7	84.3	91.0
Pakistan	4.7	6.9	4.9	7.2	71.1	78.8	74.3	83.1
Panama	7.1	12.7	7.6	13.8	83.0	87.8	88.4	92.2
Papua New Guinea	5.0	7.3	5.2	7.7	57.9	66.6	60.2	70.5
Paraguay	4.6	9.1	5.8	10.1	76.9	84.5	83.4	89.8
Peru	5.7	10.1	6.7	11.5	74.2	84.0	79.8	89.0
Philippines	4.9	8.7	5.8	10.2	69.7	79.8	76.4	86.3
Poland	12.9	19.2	18.4	25.8	74.2	81.7	89.6	92.8
Portugal	16.0	20.2	21.4	26.7	82.5	86.7	91.3	93.8
Puerto Rico	13.2	14.8	17.3	22.2	83.6	88.0	92.5	95.5

53

Table 12. The Aging Population, 1995 and 2020 (*continued*)

Economy	Population over age 60 (percentage of total)				Probability of surviving to age 60 (percentage of birth cohort)			
	Male		Female		Male		Female	
	1995	2020	1995	2020	1995	2020	1995	2020
Qatar	3.2	..	1.7	11.9	79.9	85.7	87.8	91.9
Reunion	7.5	13.6	10.2	17.6	80.0	86.9	91.6	95.1
Romania	15.4	20.3	19.4	25.5	75.2	83.5	86.2	91.2
Russian Federation	11.8	17.2	20.4	25.0	58.4	68.4	84.4	90.0
Rwanda	3.4	2.9	4.0	3.7	22.8	47.6	28.4	54.2
São Tomé and Principe	7.8	8.4	9.2	10.9	75.3	82.5	84.1	91.0
Saudi Arabia	4.1	8.4	4.5	5.5	78.8	85.3	82.1	89.3
Senegal	3.7	4.0	4.3	4.5	42.1	54.9	46.2	60.4
Seychelles	7.7	9.4	10.8	9.6	77.7	84.2	89.3	94.0
Sierra Leone	3.9	2.9	4.9	4.0	19.4	38.0	26.4	46.0
Singapore	8.5	21.4	9.7	23.7	84.9	89.1	91.1	94.2
Slovak Republic	12.7	18.4	17.4	24.1	74.7	81.7	88.7	92.2
Slovenia	13.7	24.8	20.9	30.4	80.3	87.0	91.0	94.2
Solomon Islands	4.7	4.5	4.4	5.2	65.5	74.0	68.2	79.0
Somalia	4.8	4.3	5.4	5.1	49.0	57.4	54.8	65.2
South Africa	6.0	8.3	7.0	10.5	65.1	75.9	76.8	87.6
Spain	17.5	23.3	22.5	29.6	85.7	89.0	93.4	95.7
Sri Lanka	8.2	14.0	8.5	16.9	80.3	86.7	87.6	92.1
St. Kitts and Nevis	21.1	4.2	18.2	15.4	75.6	84.0	82.9	91.6
St. Lucia	6.7	4.6	9.6	9.7	77.8	83.4	85.9	92.2
St. Vincent and the Grenadines	7.3	11.3	10.7	16.9	78.5	85.1	88.6	93.7
Sudan	4.1	5.3	4.9	6.3	47.8	64.3	53.6	69.8
Suriname	6.5	9.7	8.1	14.0	75.1	82.8	85.3	92.2
Swaziland	3.8	5.0	4.4	6.3	57.9	72.3	66.6	80.2
Sweden	19.5	25.7	24.4	29.6	88.1	90.7	93.8	95.7
Switzerland	17.3	27.7	22.6	32.8	87.4	90.3	94.0	96.2
Syrian Arab Republic	4.2	5.2	4.7	6.3	74.1	83.0	80.7	89.2
Taiwan, China	11.3	19.1	10.2	21.5	85.3	89.1	91.0	94.2
Tajikistan	5.6	7.2	7.5	9.2	75.2	81.3	84.0	89.6
Tanzania	3.7	4.1	4.4	4.6	46.8	56.0	51.9	60.5
Thailand	6.7	13.2	8.2	15.9	75.5	81.2	84.4	88.3
Togo	4.2	3.8	5.0	4.7	43.6	57.3	49.8	63.3
Tonga	7.5	7.8	7.8	10.5	74.3	83.7	82.1	91.7
Trinidad and Tobago	7.5	13.1	8.9	16.0	80.4	86.6	87.6	92.3
Tunisia	6.9	10.4	7.1	11.7	78.1	84.8	80.2	88.7
Turkey	7.6	11.7	8.2	13.0	75.5	82.2	82.7	88.8
Turkmenistan	4.8	7.7	6.8	10.1	69.3	77.0	82.4	90.3
Turks and Caicos Islands	..	..	..	..	..	..	..	..
Uganda	3.8	2.2	4.0	2.4	36.9	41.8	35.8	39.0
Ukraine	15.9	20.1	24.5	29.3	71.7	80.0	88.1	93.4
United Arab Emirates	3.0	..	2.7	12.4	85.4	89.0	89.1	92.7
United Kingdom	18.0	23.6	22.9	27.9	86.2	90.0	92.3	94.9
United States	14.1	22.0	18.7	26.3	86.3	90.5	93.0	95.5
Uruguay	15.0	16.3	18.7	22.4	79.8	86.0	89.7	94.1
Uzbekistan	5.8	8.4	7.8	11.2	76.0	82.5	86.2	92.2
Vanuatu	5.6	6.7	3.8	7.2	67.3	78.6	71.6	83.7
Venezuela	5.5	10.8	6.6	12.9	80.1	85.9	88.3	92.4
Vietnam	6.3	8.2	8.1	10.8	73.8	80.9	82.0	88.6
Virgin Islands (UK)	..	..	..	..	..	..	..	..
Virgin Islands (US)	8.3	18.4	11.8	26.4	83.9	88.6	91.6	95.0
West Bank and Gaza	..	..	..	..	..	..	..	..
Western Samoa	6.8	6.6	6.4	8.8	70.8	78.8	77.3	88.4
Yemen, Rep.	4.1	2.9	4.8	4.1	54.3	65.5	55.2	68.5
Yugoslavia, Fed. Republic	14.1	20.8	17.8	24.9	80.9	86.1	88.1	92.2
Zambia	3.8	3.6	3.8	3.9	42.1	48.1	42.8	46.9
Zimbabwe	4.2	6.1	4.6	6.6	57.0	63.1	61.2	65.5
World	8.7	12.2	10.6	14.3	72.1	79.3	78.1	85.1
Low-income	7.6	10.8	8.6	12.0	68.4	75.9	71.9	80.8
Excluding China and India	5.9	7.2	7.8	8.9	56.2	66.2	61.0	71.5
Middle-income	8.4	11.8	10.7	14.5	71.8	80.1	82.0	89.0
Low- and middle-income	7.9	11.2	9.4	12.9	69.5	77.3	75.3	83.5
East Asia and Pacific	8.4	13.4	9.2	14.8	75.6	81.6	80.7	87.2
Europe and Central Asia	11.9	17.3	15.9	21.4	69.3	77.5	86.0	91.3
Latin America and the Caribbean	7.6	10.5	9.7	13.4	74.5	81.5	84.4	89.9
Middle East and North Africa	5.6	8.0	6.1	8.8	73.1	82.3	76.2	86.3
South Asia	7.0	10.1	7.4	10.7	67.8	76.4	69.3	80.5
Sub-Saharan Africa	6.1	7.0	8.7	8.8	49.6	60.3	55.3	66.3
High-income	14.3	21.5	18.9	25.7	86.0	89.9	92.9	95.4

Table 13. Access to Safe Water, Sanitation, and Health Care

Economy	Percent of population with access to			Percent of children under 12 months with	
	Safe water 1989–95	Sanitation 1989–95	Health services 1993	Measles immunization 1995	DPT-2 immunization 1995
Afghanistan	..	..	..	19	..
Albania	..	100	..	91	97
Algeria	..	..	..	69	75
Angola	32	16	24	32	21
Anguilla	..	..	..	..	..
Antigua and Barbuda	..	..	..	..	..
Argentina	64	89	..	76	66
Armenia	..	..	..	95	83
Aruba	..	..	..	..	..
Australia	95	90	100	86	95
Austria	..	100	100	60	90
Azerbaijan	..	..	..	91	90
Bahamas, The	..	..	..	88	..
Bahrain	..	..	..	90	..
Bangladesh	83	30	74	96	91
Barbados	..	..	..	52	..
Belarus	..	100	100	96	90
Belgium	..	100	100	70	97
Belize	..	..	..	83	..
Benin	70	22	42	72	79
Bermuda	..	..	..	..	..
Bhutan	..	..	..	58	..
Bolivia	60	44	..	83	86
Bosnia and Herzegovina	..	..	..	57	67
Botswana	70	55	86	68	78
Brazil	92	73	..	78	69
Brunei	..	..	..	92	..
Bulgaria	..	99	100	93	100
Burkina Faso	..	14	..	55	47
Burundi	58	48	80	44	57
Cambodia	13	..	..	75	79
Cameroon	41	40	15	31	48
Canada	100	85	99	98	93
Cape Verde	..	..	..	95	..
Cayman Islands	..	..	..	..	..
Central African Republic	..	..	13	70	40
Chad	29	32	26	24	18
Channel Islands	..	..	..	..	..
Chile	96	71	95	93	92
China	46	..	..	89	93
Colombia	96	70	87	77	91
Comoros	..	..	..	60	..
Congo, Dem. Rep.	25	9	59	41	35
Congo, Rep.	60	9	..	39	50
Costa Rica	100	99	97	94	85
Côte d'Ivoire	..	54	60	57	40
Croatia	82	68	..	90	87
Cuba	96	66	100	100	100
Cyprus	..	..	..	83	..
Czech Republic	94	..	..	96	96
Denmark	100	100	100	88	89
Djibouti	..	..	..	68	..
Dominica	..	..	..	99	..
Dominican Republic	79	85	..	100	100
Ecuador	70	64	80	100	80
Egypt, Arab Rep.	84	..	99	82	82
El Salvador	62	73	..	94	100
Equatorial Guinea	..	..	..	70	..
Eritrea	..	..	..	45	45
Estonia	..	..	..	81	84
Ethiopia	27	10	55	54	57
Fiji	..	..	..	93	..
Finland	100	100	100	98	100
France	100	96	..	76	89
French Guiana	..	..	..	..	..
French Polynesia	..	..	..	..	..
Gabon	67	76	87	50	48
Gambia, The	61	34	..	88	93
Georgia	..	..	..	63	58
Germany	..	100	..	75	80
Ghana	56	42	25	68	71
Greece	..	96	..	70	78
Grenada	..	..	..	..	..
Guadeloupe	..	..	..	..	..
Guam	..	..	..	..	..

Table 13. Access to Safe Water, Sanitation, and Health Care (*continued*)

Economy	Percent of population with access to			Percent of children under 12 months with	
	Safe water 1989–95	Sanitation 1989–95	Health services 1993	Measles immunization 1995	DPT-2 immunization 1995
Guatemala	64	71	60	84	78
Guinea	49	6	45	69	73
Guinea-Bissau	57	20	80	68	74
Guyana	..	..	..	90	..
Haiti	28	24	45	24	30
Honduras	70	68	62	90	96
Hong Kong, China	..	..	..	42	83
Hungary	..	94	..	100	100
Iceland	..	..	..	98	..
India	63	29	..	84	92
Indonesia	63	55	43	89	91
Iran, Islamic Republic	89	82	73	95	97
Iraq	45	36	98	95	91
Ireland	..	100	..	78	65
Israel	99	70	100	94	92
Italy	..	100	..	50	50
Jamaica	70	74	..	82	93
Japan	95	85	100	68	85
Jordan	89	30	90	92	100
Kazakhstan	..	..	..	72	80
Kenya	49	43	..	73	84
Kiribati	..	..	..	89	..
Korea, Dem. Rep.	..	100	100	98	96
Korea, Rep.	89	100	100	92	93
Kuwait	..	..	100	93	100
Kyrgyz Republic	75	53	..	89	83
Lao PDR	41	30	..	65	51
Latvia	..	..	..	85	65
Lebanon	..	..	..	88	92
Lesotho	57	35	80	82	56
Liberia	..	..	..	..	..
Libya	30	18	100	89	91
Lithuania	..	..	..	94	96
Luxembourg	..	..	..	80	..
Macao	..	..	..	..	..
Macedonia, FYR	..	..	..	85	87
Madagascar	32	17	65	59	67
Malawi	54	63	80	99	98
Malaysia	90	94	88	81	90
Maldives	..	..	..	86	..
Mali	44	44	..	49	46
Malta	..	..	..	90	..
Marshall Islands	..	..	..	..	..
Martinique	..	..	..	..	..
Mauritania	72	64	..	53	50
Mauritius	100	100	99	85	89
Mayotte	..	..	..	..	..
Mexico	87	70	91	90	92
Micronesia, Fed. Sts.	..	..	..	76	..
Moldova	..	50	..	98	96
Mongolia	54	..	100	85	88
Montserrat	..	..	..	..	..
Morocco	59	63	62	92	93
Mozambique	28	23	30	71	57
Myanmar	39	42	..	66	69
Namibia	57	36	..	57	61
Nepal	48	22	..	78	77
Netherlands	100	100	100	95	97
Netherlands Antilles	..	..	..	..	..
New Caledonia	..	..	..	..	..
New Zealand	..	..	100	87	84
Nicaragua	57	..	..	81	85
Niger	57	15	30	38	19
Nigeria	43	38	67	50	44
Norway	100	100	100	93	92
Oman	56	72	89	98	99
Pakistan	60	30	85	53	55
Panama	82	87	82	84	86
Papua New Guinea	31	26	96	35	50
Paraguay	..	30	..	76	77
Peru	60	47	..	97	94
Philippines	84	75	..	86	85
Poland	..	100	100	96	95
Portugal	..	100	..	94	93
Puerto Rico	..	..	..	..	..

Table 13. Access to Safe Water, Sanitation, and Health Care (*continued*)

Economy	Percent of population with access to			Percent of children under 12 months with	
	Safe water 1989–95	Sanitation 1989–95	Health services 1993	Measles immunization 1995	DPT-2 immunization 1995
Qatar	..	..	..	87	..
Reunion	..	..	..	..	..
Romania	..	49	..	93	98
Russian Federation	..	..	..	91	72
Rwanda	..	..	..	..	..
Samoa	..	..	..	81	..
São Tomé and Principe	..	..	..	69	..
Saudi Arabia	93	86	98	94	97
Senegal	..	..	40	80	80
Seychelles	..	..	..	92	..
Sierra Leone	..	..	..	44	41
Singapore	100	100	100	88	95
Slovak Republic	..	51	..	99	99
Slovenia	..	90	..	91	98
Solomon Islands	..	..	..	76	..
Somalia	..	..	..	30	..
South Africa	..	46	..	76	73
Spain	99	97	..	90	88
Sri Lanka	57	66	90	88	91
St. Kitts and Nevis	..	..	..	100	..
St. Lucia	..	..	..	94	..
St. Vincent and the Grenadines	..	..	..	100	..
Sudan	77	55	70	74	76
Suriname	..	..	..	61	..
Swaziland	..	..	..	85	..
Sweden	..	100	100	96	99
Switzerland	100	100	100	83	89
Syrian Arab Republic	87	78	99	98	100
Taiwan, China	..	..	..	..	..
Tajikistan	..	62	..	90	95
Tanzania	49	86	93	75	79
Thailand	81	87	59	87	93
Togo	67	20	..	65	73
Tonga	..	..	..	87	..
Trinidad and Tobago	82	56	99	87	81
Tunisia	86	72	90	89	90
Turkey	92	94	100	75	86
Turkmenistan	85	60	..	90	87
Turks and Caicos Islands	..	..	..	..	..
Uganda	42	60	71	79	79
Ukraine	97	49	100	96	94
United Arab Emirates	98	95	90	90	90
United Kingdom	100	96	..	92	92
United States	90	85	..	89	94
Uruguay	34	82	..	80	86
Uzbekistan	..	18	..	71	65
Vanuatu	..	..	..	66	..
Venezuela	88	55	..	94	63
Vietnam	38	21	97	95	93
Virgin Islands (UK)	..	..	..	..	..
Virgin Islands (US)	..	..	..	..	..
West Bank and Gaza	..	..	..	..	..
Yemen, Rep.	52	51	..	49	52
Yugoslavia, Fed. Republic	..	100	..	75	79
Zambia	47	42	75	78	76
Zimbabwe	74	58	..	78	80
World	76	..	..	80	82
Low-income	53	..	..	77	80
Excluding China and India	50	31	..	65	63
Middle-income	..	..	..	86	86
Low- and middle-income	56	..	..	80	82
East Asia and Pacific	49	..	..	88	91
Europe and Central Asia	..	..	..	83	90
Latin America and the Caribbean	80	67	..	84	80
Middle East and North Africa	85	..	..	89	91
South Asia	63	29	..	80	84
Sub-Saharan Africa	47	48	..	60	58
High-income	94	92	..	83	89

Table 14. Other Health Determinants and Outcomes

Economy	Child malnutrition (% of children under five) 1990–96	Anemia (% of pregnant women) 1980–95	Low birth weight babies (% of births) 1989–95	Obesity (% obese)	Dietary energy supply (kcal/day) 1990–92	Kcal from fat (% of total calories)	Tuber-culosis incidence (per 100,000 population)	Smoking prevalence (% of adults) Male	Smoking prevalence (% of adults) Female
Afghanistan	40	..	20	..	1,660	16	278	..	..
Albania	..	..	7	..	..	..	40	50	8
Algeria	10	42	9	..	2,900	21	53	53	10
Angola	35	29	19	..	1,840	22	225	..	..
Anguilla	..	..	..	..	..	..	20	..	..
Antigua and Barbuda	10	..	8	..	..	..	20	..	..
Argentina	2	26	7	7[a]	2,950	31	50	40	23
Armenia	..	..	..	..	..	..	40	..	..
Aruba	..	..	..	..	..	..	..	..	..
Australia	..	..	..	..	..	..	6	29	21
Austria	..	..	6	..	..	..	20	42	27
Azerbaijan	10	..	..	..	..	..	47	..	..
Bahamas, The	..	12	7	..	..	..	30	19	4
Bahrain	7	..	..	..	..	..	25	24	6
Bangladesh	68	53	34	0.3[a]	1,990	8	220	60	15
Barbados	6	29	10	..	..	..	20	..	..
Belarus	..	..	5	..	..	..	50	..	..
Belgium	..	..	6	..	..	..	16	31	19
Belize	6	65	6	..	..	..	40	..	..
Benin	24	41	10	..	2,520	18	135	..	..
Bermuda	..	..	..	..	..	..	20	..	..
Bhutan	38	81	..	..	..	..	90	..	..
Bolivia	16	51	12	..	2,030	23	335	50	21
Bosnia and Herzegovina	..	..	..	..	..	..	80	..	..
Botswana	27	..	8	..	2,320	26	400	21	..
Brazil	7	33	11	5.4[a]	2,790	27	80	40	25
Brunei	..	..	..	..	..	..	70	..	..
Bulgaria	..	..	6	..	3,160	32	40	49	17
Burkina Faso	33	24	21	..	2,140	18	289	..	..
Burundi	38	68	..	1.2[a]	1,950	7	367	..	..
Cambodia	38	..	..	..	2,100	9	235	80	10
Cameroon	15	44	13	..	2,040	19	194	..	..
Canada	..	..	6	..	..	..	8	31	29
Cape Verde	19	..	..	..	..	..	100	..	..
Cayman Islands	..	..	..	..	..	..	20	..	..
Central African Republic	23	67	15	4.8[a]	1,720	29	139	..	..
Chad	..	37	..	..	..	..	167	..	..
Channel Islands	..	..	..	..	..	..	..	..	..
Chile	1	13	7	6.6[a]	2,540	23	67	38	25
China	16	52	6	4.3[a]	2,710	17	85	63	4
Colombia	8	24	9	..	2,630	21	67	35	19
Comoros	..	..	..	..	..	..	150	..	..
Congo, Dem. Rep.	34	76	15	..	2,090	15	333	..	..
Congo, Rep.	24	..	16	3.4[b]	2,210	23	250	..	..
Costa Rica	2	28	7	..	2,870	25	15	35	20
Côte d'Ivoire	24	..	14	..	2,460	17	196	..	..
Croatia	..	..	8	..	..	38	65	37	38
Cuba	8	47	8	9.5[b]	3,000	23	20	39	25
Cyprus	..	..	..	..	..	..	15	43	7
Czech Republic	1	23	6	..	..	38	25	43	31
Denmark	..	..	5	..	..	..	12	37	37
Djibouti	23	40	..	..	..	..	600	..	..
Dominica	..	28	10	..	..	..	20	..	..
Dominican Republic	6	..	16	..	2,270	26	110	66	14
Ecuador	17	17	13	..	2,540	32	166	52	28
Egypt, Arab Rep.	9	24	12	..	3,340	18	78	40	2
El Salvador	11	14	11	..	2,530	21	110	38	12
Equatorial Guinea	..	..	..	..	..	..	150	..	..
Eritrea	41	..	..	..	..	..	155	..	..
Estonia	..	..	..	..	..	..	60	52	24
Ethiopia	48	42	16	..	1,620	14	155	..	..
Fiji	8	..	..	..	..	..	40	59	31
Finland	..	..	5	..	..	..	15	27	19
France	..	..	..	..	..	..	20	40	27
French Guiana	..	..	..	..	..	..	100	..	..
French Polynesia	..	..	..	..	..	..	60	..	..
Gabon	15	..	10	..	2,490	18	100	..	..
Gambia, The	17	80	10	..	2,320	21	166	..	..
Georgia	..	..	..	..	..	..	70	45	35
Germany	..	..	..	..	..	..	18	37	22
Ghana	27	..	17	3.2[b]	2,090	15	222	10	1
Greece	..	..	9	..	..	..	12	46	28
Grenada	..	..	..	..	..	..	20	..	..
Guadeloupe	..	..	..	..	..	..	20	..	..
Guam	..	..	..	..	..	..	80	..	..

Table 14. Other Health Determinants and Outcomes (*continued*)

Economy	Child malnutrition (% of children under five) 1990–96	Anemia (% of pregnant women) 1980–95	Low birth weight babies (% of births) 1989–95	Obesity (% obese)	Dietary energy supply (kcal/day) 1990–92	Kcal from fat (% of total calories)	Tuberculosis incidence (per 100,000 population)	Smoking prevalence (% of adults) Male	Smoking prevalence (% of adults) Female
Guatemala	33	39	14	2.8[a]	2,280	17	110	38	18
Guinea	24	..	21	..	2,400	18	166	40	2
Guinea-Bissau	23	74	20	..	..	..	220	..	..
Guyana	18	..	18	2.3[a]	2,350	14	50	..	..
Haiti	28	38	15	..	1,740	13	333	..	..
Honduras	18	..	9	1.8[a]	2,310	24	133	36	11
Hong Kong, China	..	..	..	..	..	..	140	..	..
Hungary	..	..	9	..	3,560	39	50	44	27
Iceland	..	..	..	..	..	..	10	31	28
India	66	88	33	0.5[b]	2,330	..	220	40	3
Indonesia	40	64	14	..	2,700	17	220	53	4
Iran, Islamic Republic	16	..	12	..	2,760	21	50	..	..
Iraq	12	18	15	..	2,270	17	150	40	5
Ireland	..	..	4	..	..	..	18	29	28
Israel	..	..	..	..	..	..	12	45	30
Italy	..	..	..	..	..	..	25	38	26
Jamaica	10	40	11	..	2,580	22	10	43	13
Japan	3	..	6	..	..	..	42	59	15
Jordan	10	..	7	..	2,900	25	14	48	9
Kazakhstan	1	11	..	15[a]	..	..	77	..	..
Kenya	23	35	16	2.4[b]	1,970	21	140	52	7
Kiribati	..	..	..	..	..	..	400	..	..
Korea, Dem. Rep.	..	..	..	..	2,930	..	162	..	..
Korea, Rep.	..	..	4	..	3,270	..	162	68	7
Kuwait	6	40	..	..	2,460	32	40	52	12
Kyrgyz Republic	..	..	..	..	..	..	68	48	15
Lao PDR	40	..	18	0.7[b]	2,210	14	235	41	15
Latvia	..	..	..	..	..	..	70	67	12
Lebanon	9	..	..	..	3,260	27	35	..	..
Lesotho	21	7	11	..	2,260	14	250	38	1
Liberia	20	78	..	..	1,780	20	100	..	..
Libya	5	..	5	..	3,290	30	12	..	..
Lithuania	..	..	..	..	..	..	82	52	10
Luxembourg	..	..	..	..	..	..	10	32	26
Macao	..	..	..	..	..	..	100	..	..
Macedonia, FYR	..	..	..	..	..	24	60	..	..
Madagascar	32	..	10	..	2,160	13	310	29	28
Malawi	28	55	20	..	1,910	11	173	..	..
Malaysia	23	56	8	..	2,830	32	67	41	4
Maldives	39	20	..	..	..	..	120	..	..
Mali	31	58	17	0.5[a]	2,230	17	289	..	..
Malta	..	..	..	..	..	..	10	40	18
Marshall Islands	..	..	..	..	..	..	150	..	..
Martinique	..	..	..	..	..	..	20	..	..
Mauritania	48	..	11	..	2,610	21	220	..	..
Mauritius	15	29	8	5.6[b]	2,780	24	50	47	4
Mayotte	..	..	..	..	..	..	..	..	..
Mexico	14	14	12	..	3,190	27	60	38	14
Micronesia, Fed. Sts.	..	..	..	..	..	..	60	..	..
Moldova	..	50	..	..	..	..	70	..	..
Mongolia	12	45	10	..	2,100	33	100	40	7
Montserrat	..	..	..	..	..	..	20	..	..
Morocco	10	45	9	5.2[a]	3,000	17	125	40	9
Mozambique	47	58	20	..	1,740	19	189	..	..
Myanmar	31	58	16	..	2,580	15	189	..	..
Namibia	26	16	12	..	2,190	14	400	..	..
Nepal	49	65	26	..	2,140	12	167	..	..
Netherlands	..	..	..	..	..	..	13	36	29
Netherlands Antilles	..	..	..	..	..	..	20	..	..
New Caledonia	..	..	..	..	..	..	90	..	..
New Zealand	..	..	6	..	..	..	10	24	22
Nicaragua	24	36	15	..	2,290	20	110	..	..
Niger	43	41	15	..	2,190	13	144	41	26
Nigeria	35	55	16	..	2,100	21	222	24	7
Norway	..	..	5	..	..	..	8	36	36
Oman	14	54	10	..	..	..	20	..	..
Pakistan	40	37	25	..	2,340	24	150	27	4
Panama	7	..	10	..	2,240	26	90	56	20
Papua New Guinea	30	13	23	1.6[a]	2,610	21	275	46	28
Paraguay	4	29	8	..	2,620	32	166	24	6
Peru	11	..	11	9[b]	1,880	16	250	41	13
Philippines	30	48	..	0.9[a]	2,290	15	400	43	8
Poland	..	16	8	..	3,340	32	50	51	29
Portugal	..	..	5	..	..	..	60	38	15
Puerto Rico	..	..	..	..	..	..	8	..	..

Table 14. Other Health Determinants and Outcomes (*continued*)

Economy	Child malnutrition (% of children under five) 1990–96	Anemia (% of pregnant women) 1980–95	Low birth weight babies (% of births) 1989–95	Obesity (% obese)	Dietary energy supply (kcal/day) 1990–92	Kcal from fat (% of total calories)	Tuberculosis incidence (per 100,000 population)	Smoking prevalence (% of adults) Male	Smoking prevalence (% of adults) Female
Qatar	6	..	..	..	..	..	50	..	..
Reunion	..	..	..	..	..	..	..	..	..
Romania	6	31	..	..	3,160	34	120	43	15
Russian Federation	3	30	..	..	..	..	99	67	30
Rwanda	29	..	17	..	1,860	8	260	..	..
Samoa	..	..	..	..	..	..	30	..	..
São Tomé and Principe	17	..	..	..	..	..	100	..	..
Saudi Arabia	..	..	..	..	..	..	22	53	..
Senegal	22	26	11	3.7[b]	2,310	23	166	48	35
Seychelles	6	..	..	..	..	..	40	..	..
Sierra Leone	29	..	17	..	1,820	28	167	..	..
Singapore	14	..	7	..	..	..	82	32	3
Slovak Republic	..	..	6	..	..	..	40	43	26
Slovenia	..	..	6	..	..	37	35	35	23
Solomon Islands	21	..	..	..	..	..	120	..	..
Somalia	39	78	16	..	1,590	28	222	..	..
South Africa	9	37	..	..	2,810	22	250	52	17
Spain	..	..	..	..	..	..	49	48	25
Sri Lanka	38	39	17	0.1[a]	2,230	18	167	55	1
St. Kitts and Nevis	..	..	..	..	..	..	25	..	..
St. Lucia	..	..	..	..	..	..	20	..	..
St. Vincent and the Grenadines	..	..	..	..	..	..	25	..	..
Sudan	34	36	15	..	2,150	26	211	..	..
Suriname	..	..	..	..	..	..	100	..	..
Swaziland	10	..	..	..	2,680	18	200	33	8
Sweden	..	..	5	..	..	..	7	22	24
Switzerland	..	..	5	..	..	..	18	36	26
Syrian Arab Republic	..	..	8	..	..	..	58	..	..
Taiwan, China	..	..	..	..	..	..	..	..	..
Tajikistan	..	50	..	..	..	..	133	..	..
Tanzania	29	..	14	..	2,110	13	187	..	..
Thailand	13	57	13	1.3[a]	2,380	17	173	49	4
Togo	25	48	20	2.5[a]	2,290	18	244	..	..
Tonga	..	..	..	..	..	..	40	65	14
Trinidad and Tobago	7	53	10	3.3[a]	2,630	25	20	42	8
Tunisia	9	..	10	3.8[a]	3,260	25	55	58	6
Turkey	10	..	8	..	..	..	57	63	24
Turkmenistan	..	..	..	..	..	24	72	27	1
Turks and Caicos Islands	..	..	..	..	..	..	20	..	..
Uganda	26	30	..	2.4[a]	2,220	11	300	10	0
Ukraine	..	..	5	..	..	..	50	50	47
United Arab Emirates	7	46	..	..	3,370	30	30	..	..
United Kingdom	..	..	..	..	..	..	12	28	26
United States	..	..	7	..	..	..	10	28	23
Uruguay	4	20	8	..	2,680	32	20	41	27
Uzbekistan	4	..	..	7.8[a]	..	..	55	49	9
Vanuatu	..	..	..	..	..	..	120	..	..
Venezuela	5	29	9	3.3[a]	2,590	26	44	..	..
Vietnam	45	52.3	17	..	2,200	12	166	73	4
Virgin Islands (UK)	..	..	..	..	..	..	20	..	..
Virgin Islands (US)	..	..	..	..	..	..	20	..	..
West Bank and Gaza	..	..	..	..	..	..	..	..	..
Yemen, Rep.	30	..	19	..	2,160	..	96	..	..
Yugoslavia, Fed. Republic	..	..	..	..	..	..	50	52	31
Zambia	29	34	13	5.7[b]	2,020	13	345	39	7
Zimbabwe	16	..	14	4.4[a]	2,080	23	207	36	15
World	30	..	..	..	..	..	..	..	..
Low-income	..	..	..	..	..	..	..	..	..
Excluding China and India	..	..	..	..	..	..	..	..	..
Middle-income	..	..	..	..	..	..	..	..	..
Low- and middle-income	32	..	..	..	..	..	..	..	..
East Asia and Pacific	23	..	..	..	..	..	..	..	..
Europe and Central Asia	3	..	..	..	..	..	..	..	..
Latin America and the Caribbean	11	..	..	..	..	..	..	..	..
Middle East and North Africa	16	..	..	..	..	..	..	..	..
South Asia	52	..	..	..	..	..	..	..	..
Sub-Saharan Africa	30	..	..	..	..	..	..	..	..
High-income	..	..	..	..	..	..	..	..	..

a. Children's obesity.
b. Adults' obesity.

Table 15. Reproductive Health Indicators

Economy	Maternal mortality ratio (per 100,000 live births) 1990–95	Adolescent fertility rate (per 1,000 15–19 yr. olds) 1995	Contraceptive prevalence rate (% of married women) 1990–95	Adult HIV prevalence (% of over-15 population) 1994–95	Births attended by health staff (%) 1990–96
Afghanistan	1700	153	..	0.0	9
Albania	23	26	..	0.0	99
Algeria	140	17	51	0.1	77
Angola	1500	218	..	1.0	15
Anguilla	..	..	..	..	..
Antigua and Barbuda	..	57	..	..	..
Argentina	140	62	..	0.4	97
Armenia	35	50	..	0.0	..
Aruba	..	..	..	..	..
Australia	9	31	..	0.1	100
Austria	10	23	..	0.2	100
Azerbaijan	29	33	..	0.0	..
Bahamas, The	100	56	..	3.9	..
Bahrain	60	27	..	0.2	..
Bangladesh	887	116	40	0.0	14
Barbados	43	50	..	2.8	..
Belarus	25	39	..	0.0	..
Belgium	10	11	..	0.2	100
Belize	..	92	..	2.0	..
Benin	990	127	..	1.2	45
Bermuda	..	..	..	..	..
Bhutan	..	67	..	0.0	15
Bolivia	373	82	45	0.1	47
Bosnia and Herzegovina	..	28	..	0.0	..
Botswana	220	106	..	18.0	78
Brazil	200	37	..	0.7	81
Brunei	60	28	..	0.2	..
Bulgaria	20	60	..	0.0	86
Burkina Faso	939	149	8	6.7	42
Burundi	1327	66	..	2.7	19
Cambodia	900	108	..	1.9	47
Cameroon	550	136	16	3.0	64
Canada	6	25	..	0.2	99
Cape Verde	..	26	..	..	..
Cayman Islands	..	..	..	..	..
Central African Republic	649	145	15	5.8	46
Chad	1594	183	..	2.7	15
Channel Islands	..	21	..	..	..
Chile	65	48	..	0.1	98
China	115	17	83	0.0	84
Colombia	107	80	72	0.2	85
Comoros	950	131	..	0.1	..
Congo, Dem. Rep.	870	221	..	3.7	..
Congo, Rep.	822	140	..	7.2	..
Costa Rica	55	67	75	0.5	93
Côte d'Ivoire	887	136	11	6.8	45
Croatia	10	28	..	0.0	..
Cuba	36	68	..	0.0	90
Cyprus	5	34	..	0.3	..
Czech Republic	12	34	69	0.0	..
Denmark	9	18	..	0.2	100
Djibouti	570	171	..	3.0	..
Dominica	..	47	..	..	..
Dominican Republic	110	53	56	1.0	92
Ecuador	150	68	57	0.3	64
Egypt, Arab Rep.	170	56	47	0.0	46
El Salvador	300	91	53	0.6	87
Equatorial Guinea	820	182	..	1.1	..
Eritrea	1400	125	..	3.2	21
Estonia	41	36	..	0.0	..
Ethiopia	1528	164	4	2.5	14
Fiji	90	43	..	0.0	..
Finland	11	20	..	0.0	100
France	15	17	..	0.3	99
French Guiana	..	..	..	..	..
French Polynesia	..	51	..	..	..
Gabon	483	150	..	2.3	80
Gambia, The	1050	167	12	2.1	44
Georgia	55	40	..	0.0	..
Germany	22	14	..	0.1	99
Ghana	742	109	20	2.3	44
Greece	10	19	..	0.1	97
Grenada	..	59	..	..	..
Guadeloupe	..	34	..	..	..
Guam	..	58	..	..	..

Table 15. Reproductive Health Indicators (*continued*)

Economy	Maternal mortality ratio (per 100,000 live births) 1990–95	Adolescent fertility rate (per 1,000 15–19 yr. olds) 1995	Contraceptive prevalence rate (% of married women) 1990–95	Adult HIV prevalence (% of over-15 population) 1994–95	Births attended by health staff (%) 1990–96
Guatemala	464	106	31	0.4	35
Guinea	880	213	..	0.6	31
Guinea-Bissau	910	186	..	3.1	27
Guyana	..	56	..	1.3	..
Haiti	600	70	18	4.4	21
Honduras	220	112	47	1.6	88
Hong Kong, China	7	13	..	0.1	100
Hungary	10	31	..	0.1	99
Iceland	0	29	..	0.1	..
India	437	81	43	0.4	34
Indonesia	390	57	55	0.0	36
Iran, Islamic Republic	120	80	..	0.0	77
Iraq	310	61	..	0.0	54
Ireland	10	23	60	0.1	..
Israel	7	28	..	0.1	99
Italy	12	14	..	0.3	..
Jamaica	120	67	67	0.9	82
Japan	18	6	..	0.0	100
Jordan	132	43	35	0.0	87
Kazakhstan	53	40	59	0.0	99
Kenya	650	95	33	8.3	45
Kiribati	..	54	..	..	..
Korea, Dem. Rep.	48	30	..	0.0	100
Korea, Rep.	30	8	79	0.0	98
Kuwait	18	45	..	0.1	99
Kyrgyz Republic	80	44	..	0.0	..
Lao PDR	660	59	..	0.0	..
Latvia	40	34	..	0.0	..
Lebanon	300	43	..	0.1	45
Lesotho	598	55	23	3.1	40
Liberia	560	211	..	1.3	58
Libya	220	106	..	0.1	76
Lithuania	16	34	..	0.0	100
Luxembourg	0	16	..	0.1	..
Macao	..	15	..	..	..
Macedonia, FYR	12	38	..	0.0	..
Madagascar	660	145	17	0.1	57
Malawi	620	151	13	13.6	55
Malaysia	34	30	..	0.3	94
Maldives	..	76	..	0.1	..
Mali	1249	190	..	1.3	24
Malta	0	13	..	0.1	..
Marshall Islands	..	..	..	..	..
Martinique	..	32	..	..	..
Mauritania	800	123	4	0.7	40
Mauritius	112	42	75	0.1	97
Mayotte	..	..	..	..	..
Mexico	110	57	..	0.4	77
Micronesia, Fed. Sts.	..	51	..	..	..
Moldova	34	46	..	0.0	..
Mongolia	240	45	..	0.0	99
Montserrat	..	62	..	..	..
Morocco	372	38	50	0.0	40
Mozambique	1512	122	..	5.8	25
Myanmar	518	30	..	1.5	57
Namibia	370	130	29	6.5	68
Nepal	515	82	23	0.1	7
Netherlands	12	8	..	0.0	100
Netherlands Antilles	..	33	..	..	..
New Caledonia	..	47	..	..	..
New Zealand	25	43	..	0.1	99
Nicaragua	160	136	44	0.1	61
Niger	593	222	4	1.0	15
Nigeria	1000	120	6	2.2	31
Norway	6	22	..	0.1	100
Oman	190	123	9	0.1	87
Pakistan	340	107	12	0.1	19
Panama	55	61	..	0.6	100
Papua New Guinea	930	44	..	0.2	20
Paraguay	180	72	48	0.1	66
Peru	280	52	59	0.2	52
Philippines	208	47	40	0.1	53
Poland	10	28	..	0.1	99
Portugal	15	23	..	0.2	90
Puerto Rico	21	48	..	..	..

Table 15. Reproductive Health Indicators (*continued*)

Economy	Maternal mortality ratio (per 100,000 live births) 1990–95	Adolescent fertility rate (per 1,000 15–19 yr. olds) 1995	Contraceptive prevalence rate (% of married women) 1990–95	Adult HIV prevalence (% of over-15 population) 1994–95	Births attended by health staff (%) 1990–96
Qatar	..	40	..	0.1	..
Reunion	..	51	..	0.0	..
Romania	48	34	57	0.0	100
Russian Federation	52	31	..	0.0	..
Rwanda	1512	65	21	7.2	26
Samoa	35	42	..	..	..
São Tomé and Principe	..	149	..	..	..
Saudi Arabia	18	61	..	0.0	82
Senegal	510	118	7	1.4	46
Seychelles	..	51	..	..	..
Sierra Leone	800	203	..	3.0	25
Singapore	10	13	..	0.1	100
Slovak Republic	8	35	..	0.0	..
Slovenia	5	19	..	0.0	..
Solomon Islands	..	94	..	..	..
Somalia	1600	191	..	0.3	2
South Africa	404	68	..	3.2	82
Spain	7	11	..	0.6	96
Sri Lanka	30	33	..	0.1	..
St. Kitts and Nevis	..	68	..	..	..
St. Lucia	..	84	..	..	..
St. Vincent and the Grenadines	..	52	..	..	..
Sudan	660	84	9	1.0	69
Suriname	..	52	..	1.2	..
Swaziland	560	111	..	3.8	..
Sweden	7	20	..	0.1	100
Switzerland	6	7	..	0.3	99
Syrian Arab Republic	179	89	..	0.0	67
Taiwan, China	..	24	..	..	..
Tajikistan	39	48	..	0.0	..
Tanzania	748	123	10	6.4	53
Thailand	200	18	..	2.1	71
Togo	626	124	..	8.5	54
Tonga	..	32	..	..	..
Trinidad and Tobago	90	46	..	0.9	98
Tunisia	139	32	..	0.0	69
Turkey	183	44	63	0.0	76
Turkmenistan	43	26	..	0.0	..
Turks and Caicos Islands	..	..	..	..	..
Uganda	506	193	15	14.5	..
Ukraine	33	48	..	0.0	100
United Arab Emirates	33	58	..	0.2	94
United Kingdom	20	30	..	0.1	100
United States	12	60	..	0.5	99
Uruguay	85	47	..	0.3	96
Uzbekistan	43	43	..	0.0	..
Vanuatu	280	55	..	..	..
Venezuela	200	60	..	0.3	69
Vietnam	105	42	49	0.1	95
Virgin Islands (UK)	..	..	..	..	..
Virgin Islands (US)	..	74	..	..	..
West Bank and Gaza	..	..	..	..	..
Yemen, Rep.	1471	141	..	0.0	16
Yugoslavia, Fed. Republic	..	41	..	0.1	..
Zambia	230	122	15	17.1	51
Zimbabwe	570	68	48	17.4	69
World	..	..	..	0.6	..
Low-income	..	..	..	0.8	..
Excluding China and India	..	..	..	2.3	..
Middle-income	..	..	..	0.3	..
Low- and middle-income	..	..	..	0.6	..
East Asia and Pacific	..	..	..	0.1	..
Europe and Central Asia	..	..	..	0.0	..
Latin America and the Caribbean	..	..	..	0.5	..
Middle East and North Africa	..	..	..	0.0	..
South Asia	..	..	..	0.3	..
Sub-Saharan Africa	..	..	..	4.3	..
High-income	..	..	..	0.3	..

Table 16. Burden of Disease, 1990

Cause	EME	FSE	India	China	OAI	SSA	LAC	MEC	World	MDC	LDC
					Percentage of total DALYs[a]						
Total DALYs (1,000)	98,794	62,200	287,739	208,407	177,671	295,294	98,285	150,849	1,379,238	160,994	1,218,244
Communicable, maternal, perinatal, and nutritional conditions	7.1	8.8	56.4	24.2	44.7	65.9	35.3	47.7	43.9	7.8	48.7
Infectious and parasitic diseases	2.8	2.7	28.9	7.5	22.3	42.5	17.6	20.2	22.9	2.7	25.6
Tuberculosis	0.1	0.6	4.8	2.0	3.1	3.4	1.8	1.7	2.8	0.3	3.1
STDs, excluding HIV	0.4	0.6	1.9	0.1	2.3	2.1	1.2	0.5	1.4	0.5	1.5
HIV	1.3	0.1	0.1	0.0	0.1	2.8	1.1	0.0	0.8	0.8	0.8
Diarrheal diseases	0.2	0.4	10.2	1.8	7.7	10.9	5.5	9.8	7.2	0.3	8.1
Childhood-cluster diseases	0.0	0.1	6.4	1.1	4.5	10.3	3.4	5.7	5.2	0.0	5.8
Bacterial meningitis and meningococcaemia	0.2	0.4	0.5	0.6	0.5	0.3	0.5	0.5	0.5	0.3	0.5
Malaria	0.0	0.0	0.4	0.0	1.4	9.2	0.5	0.3	2.3	0.0	2.6
Tropical cluster diseases and leprosy	0.0	0.0	1.2	0.1	0.4	1.9	0.8	0.2	0.8	0.0	0.0
Intestinal nematode infections	0.0	0.0	0.3	0.7	0.9	0.2	0.7	0.1	0.4	0.0	0.4
Other infectious and parasitic diseases	0.5	0.6	3.1	1.2	1.5	1.4	2.1	1.4	1.7	0.5	2.7
Respiratory infections	1.4	2.0	11.9	5.9	8.7	10.5	4.9	10.7	8.5	1.6	9.4
Lower respiratory infections	1.2	1.9	11.4	5.7	8.5	10.2	4.7	10.4	8.2	1.5	9.1
Other respiratory infections	0.1	0.1	0.5	0.2	0.3	0.2	0.2	0.3	0.3	0.1	0.3
Maternal conditions	0.3	0.9	2.6	1.3	2.3	3.2	1.7	2.4	2.2	0.6	2.4
Obstructed labor	0.2	0.2	0.5	0.3	0.5	0.6	0.4	0.7	0.5	0.2	0.5
Abortion	0.0	0.3	0.6	0.0	0.4	0.6	0.5	0.2	0.4	0.1	0.4
Other maternal conditions	0.1	0.4	1.5	0.9	1.3	2.1	0.9	1.5	1.3	0.2	1.5
Perinatal conditions	1.8	2.2	8.8	4.9	6.9	6.5	7.4	9.7	6.7	1.9	7.3
Nutritional deficiencies	0.9	1.0	4.2	4.6	4.4	3.2	3.7	4.7	3.7	0.9	4.1
Protein-energy malnutrition	0.1	0.2	1.8	1.0	1.7	1.8	1.7	2.4	1.5	0.1	1.7
Vitamin A deficiency	0.0	0.0	0.4	0.4	0.5	0.4	0.3	0.7	0.4	0.0	0.4
Iodine deficiency	0.7	0.7	2.1	3.2	2.3	0.9	1.7	1.6	1.8	0.7	1.9
Other nutritional deficiencies	0.0	0.1	0.0	0.0	0.0	0.0	0.0	0.0	0.0	0.1	0.0
Noncommunicable	81.0	72.6	29.0	58.2	40.9	18.8	48.2	39.3	40.9	77.7	36.1
Malignant neoplasms	15.0	11.7	2.5	8.7	5.1	2.1	4.5	2.4	5.1	13.7	4.0
Stomach cancer	1.1	1.6	0.2	1.6	0.4	0.1	0.4	0.2	0.6	1.3	0.5
Colon and rectal cancers	1.6	1.1	0.1	0.5	0.3	0.1	0.2	0.1	0.3	1.4	0.2
Liver cancer	0.3	0.3	0.1	1.9	0.5	0.3	0.1	0.1	0.5	0.3	0.5
Trachea, bronchial, and lung cancers	3.0	2.6	0.1	1.0	0.5	0.1	0.3	0.2	0.6	2.8	0.4
Breast cancer	1.4	0.8	0.2	0.2	0.3	0.1	0.4	0.1	0.3	1.2	0.2
Cervix uteri cancer	0.2	0.3	0.3	0.1	0.3	0.1	0.4	0.1	0.2	0.2	0.2
Lymphomas and multiple myelomas	0.7	0.4	0.1	0.2	0.2	0.2	0.3	0.1	0.2	0.6	0.2
Leukemia	0.6	0.5	0.1	0.8	0.5	0.1	0.3	0.2	0.3	0.6	0.3
Other malignant neoplasms	6.0	4.1	1.3	2.4	2.2	1.1	2.0	1.2	2.0	5.3	1.6
Diabetes mellitus	2.4	1.1	0.8	0.5	0.7	0.2	1.5	1.0	0.8	1.9	0.7
Neuropsychiatric conditions	25.0	17.2	7.0	14.2	10.8	4.0	15.9	8.7	10.5	22.0	9.0
Unipolar major depression	6.8	5.0	2.8	6.2	3.8	1.5	4.3	3.0	3.7	6.1	3.4
Bipolar disorder	1.7	1.3	0.8	1.8	1.1	0.4	1.2	0.9	1.0	1.6	1.0
Schizophrenia	2.3	1.4	0.6	1.3	1.3	0.2	1.3	0.9	0.9	1.9	0.8
Alcohol use	4.7	2.8	0.3	0.7	1.1	0.6	3.9	0.2	1.2	4.0	0.8
Dementia and other CNS disorders	2.9	1.5	0.3	0.7	0.5	0.1	0.6	0.2	0.6	2.4	0.4
Drug use	1.5	0.9	0.0	0.1	0.5	0.1	1.1	0.6	0.4	1.3	0.3
Epilepsy	0.5	0.6	0.3	0.4	0.5	0.2	0.7	0.3	0.4	0.5	0.4
Other neuropsychiatric conditions	4.6	3.7	1.8	2.9	2.1	0.9	2.8	2.5	2.2	4.2	2.0
Glaucoma and cataracts	0.1	0.1	1.0	1.0	0.9	0.7	0.6	0.6	0.8	0.1	0.8
Cardiovascular diseases	18.6	23.2	8.1	11.0	10.1	3.9	7.9	11.1	9.7	20.4	8.2
Rheumatic heart disease	0.2	0.6	0.5	1.1	0.1	0.2	0.2	0.5	0.4	0.3	0.5
Ischemic heart disease	9.0	11.4	3.5	2.9	2.2	0.8	3.0	3.5	3.4	9.9	2.5
Cerebrovascular disease	5.0	7.2	1.5	5.2	2.5	1.6	2.5	1.6	2.8	5.9	2.4
Inflammatory heart diseases	0.7	0.7	0.6	0.6	1.3	0.5	0.5	1.2	0.7	0.7	0.8
Other cardiovascular diseases	3.7	3.3	2.0	1.1	4.0	0.9	1.7	4.2	2.3	3.6	2.1
Respiratory disease	4.8	4.8	2.6	10.7	2.7	2.6	4.0	4.2	4.4	4.8	4.3
Chronic obstructive pulmonary disease	2.3	1.7	0.9	8.5	0.7	0.6	1.0	0.9	2.1	2.1	2.1
Asthma	1.3	0.8	0.5	1.3	0.8	0.5	1.0	0.6	0.8	1.1	0.7
Other respiratory diseases	1.3	2.2	1.3	0.8	1.2	1.5	2.0	2.7	1.5	1.6	1.5
Digestive diseases	4.4	4.4	2.2	4.9	4.7	1.8	3.8	4.2	3.4	4.4	3.3
Cirrhosis of the liver	1.6	1.2	1.0	1.5	1.3	0.2	1.2	0.5	1.0	1.5	0.9
Other digestive diseases	2.8	3.2	1.2	3.4	3.4	1.6	2.6	3.7	2.5	2.9	2.4
Musculo-skeletal diseases	4.2	4.4	0.5	1.7	1.2	0.4	3.1	0.6	1.4	4.3	1.0
Rheumatoid arthritis	0.9	0.8	0.1	0.3	0.1	0.0	0.6	0.1	0.2	0.9	0.2
Osteoarthritis	2.7	3.2	0.4	1.0	0.9	0.3	2.1	0.4	1.0	2.9	0.7
Other musculo-skeletal diseases	0.5	0.4	0.0	0.3	0.2	0.0	0.4	0.1	0.2	0.5	0.1
Congential abnormalities	2.2	2.2	2.9	3.0	2.3	1.3	2.7	2.7	2.4	2.2	2.4
Oral conditions	0.9	0.8	0.4	0.5	0.7	0.1	1.0	0.9	0.5	0.8	0.5
Other noncommunicable diseases	3.4	2.8	0.9	2.1	1.7	1.6	3.3	2.9	2.0	3.2	1.8

Table 16. Burden of Disease, 1990 (*continued*)

Cause	EME	FSE	India	China	OAI	SSA	LAC	MEC	World	MDC	LDC
					Percentage of total DALYs[a]						
Injuries	11.9	18.7	14.6	17.6	14.4	15.4	16.4	13.0	15.1	14.5	15.2
Unintentional	8.7	12.9	13.0	12.9	12.1	9.3	11.0	6.8	11.0	10.3	11.1
Road-trafffic accidents	4.4	4.4	2.1	2.1	2.7	1.9	4.1	1.7	2.5	4.4	2.2
Poisoning	0.3	1.5	0.3	0.7	0.6	0.4	0.2	0.2	0.5	0.7	0.4
Falls	1.4	1.8	3.5	2.2	2.3	0.7	1.7	1.1	1.9	1.5	2.0
Fires	0.3	0.3	2.0	0.3	0.3	1.2	0.3	0.5	0.9	0.3	0.9
Drowning	0.3	1.0	0.9	2.1	1.6	1.1	0.9	0.6	1.1	0.5	1.2
Other unintentional injuries	2.2	3.9	4.2	5.5	4.7	4.0	4.8	2.7	4.1	2.8	4.3
Intentional injuries	3.2	5.8	1.5	4.7	2.3	6.0	4.5	6.2	4.1	4.2	4.1
Self-inflicted injuries	2.2	2.6	1.0	3.9	1.1	0.2	0.6	0.9	1.4	2.3	1.2
Violence	1.0	1.4	0.5	0.8	0.9	2.2	3.2	0.8	1.3	1.1	1.3
War	0.0	1.8	0.0	0.0	0.3	3.6	0.7	4.5	1.5	0.7	1.5
Other intentional injuries	0.0	0.0	0.0	0.0	0.0	0.0	0.0	0.0	0.0	0.0	0.0

EME: Established market economies.
FSE: Formerly socialist economies of Europe.
IOAI: Other Asia and islands (Asia, excluding Japan and Central Asia; Oceania, excluding Australia and New Zealand; and Indian Ocean islands).
SSA: Sub-Saharan Africa.
LAC: Latin America and the Caribbean.
MEC: Middle Eastern Crescent.
MDC: More-developed countries.
LDC: Less-developed countries.
a. DALYs are disability-adjusted life-years.

Table 17. Burden of Disease, 2020

Cause	EME	FSE	India	China	OAI	SSA	LAC	MEC	World	MDC	LDC
Total DALYs (1,000)	97,000	63,534	236,741	220,667	165,978	329,566	107,639	167,710	1,388,836	160,534	1,228,302
Communicable, maternal, perinatal, and nutritional conditions	5.2	3.0	24.4	4.3	16.5	39.8	12.6	19.9	20.1	4.3	22.2
Infectious and parasitic diseases	1.9	1.0	17.3	1.4	9.7	28.5	7.4	8.4	12.9	2.1	14.3
Tuberculosis	0.1	0.1	6.7	0.4	1.2	6.7	0.5	0.5	3.1	0.1	3.4
STDs, excluding HIV	0.2	0.2	0.7	0.0	0.9	1.0	0.4	0.2	0.6	0.2	0.6
HIV	2.3	0.2	4.6	0.1	3.0	4.4	2.9	0.2	2.6	1.5	2.8
Diarrheal diseases	0.1	0.1	2.5	0.3	2.2	5.5	1.5	4.2	2.7	0.1	3.0
Childhood-cluster diseases	0.0	0.0	1.5	0.2	1.2	5.1	0.9	2.4	2.0	0.0	2.3
Bacterial meningitis and meningococcaemia	0.1	0.1	0.1	0.1	0.1	0.2	0.1	0.2	0.1	0.1	0.1
Malaria	0.0	0.0	0.1	0.0	0.3	4.5	0.1	0.1	1.1	0.0	1.3
Tropical cluster diseases and leprosy	0.0	0.0	0.2	0.0	0.1	0.5	0.2	0.1	0.2	0.0	0.0
Intestinal nematode infections	0.0	0.0	0.1	0.1	0.2	0.1	0.2	0.0	0.1	0.0	0.1
Other infectious and parasitic diseases	0.2	0.2	0.7	0.2	0.4	0.6	0.5	0.6	0.5	0.2	0.7
Respiratory infections	1.2	0.8	3.2	1.1	2.8	5.4	1.5	4.6	3.2	1.0	3.4
Lower respiratory infections	1.1	0.8	3.1	1.1	2.8	5.3	1.5	4.5	3.1	1.0	3.3
Other respiratory infections	0.1	0.0	0.1	0.0	0.1	0.1	0.0	0.1	0.1	0.0	0.1
Maternal conditions	0.0	0.1	0.3	0.1	0.3	0.6	0.2	0.4	0.3	0.1	0.3
Obstructed labor	0.0	0.0	0.1	0.0	0.1	0.1	0.1	0.1	0.1	0.0	0.1
Abortion	0.0	0.0	0.1	0.0	0.1	0.1	0.1	0.0	0.1	0.0	0.1
Other maternal conditions	0.0	0.1	0.2	0.0	0.2	0.4	0.1	0.3	0.2	0.0	0.2
Perinatal conditions	0.7	0.7	2.4	0.9	2.2	3.7	2.3	4.6	2.5	0.7	2.7
Nutritional deficiencies	0.4	0.3	1.2	0.9	1.4	1.5	1.1	1.9	1.2	0.4	1.3
Protein-energy malnutrition	0.0	0.1	0.4	0.2	0.5	1.0	0.5	1.0	0.6	0.0	0.6
Vitamin A deficiency	0.0	0.0	0.1	0.1	0.1	0.2	0.1	0.2	0.1	0.0	0.1
Iodine deficiency	0.3	0.2	0.6	0.7	0.8	0.4	0.5	0.6	0.5	0.3	0.6
Other nutritional deficiencies	0.0	0.0	0.0	0.0	0.0	0.0	0.0	0.0	0.0	0.0	0.0
Noncommunicable	84.7	79.7	56.5	79.3	66.3	31.9	68.1	59.6	59.7	82.7	56.7
Malignant neoplasms	17.3	16.1	7.1	18.7	11.6	4.5	8.5	5.3	9.9	16.8	9.0
Stomach cancer	1.2	2.4	0.5	3.7	1.0	0.3	0.8	0.4	1.2	1.7	1.1
Colon and rectal cancers	1.9	1.4	0.2	1.0	0.6	0.1	0.5	0.2	0.6	1.7	0.4
Liver cancer	0.4	0.4	0.1	4.2	1.3	0.7	0.1	0.2	1.1	0.4	1.2
Trachea, bronchial, and lung cancers	4.6	4.4	1.5	3.4	1.9	0.2	1.3	1.2	1.8	4.5	1.5
Breast cancer	1.3	0.8	0.4	0.3	0.5	0.2	0.8	0.3	0.4	1.1	0.4
Cervix uteri cancer	0.2	0.3	0.6	0.2	0.6	0.3	0.7	0.2	0.4	0.2	0.4
Lymphomas and multiple myelomas	0.7	0.5	0.2	0.3	0.4	0.4	0.4	0.2	0.4	0.6	0.3
Leukemia	0.6	0.5	0.2	0.9	0.6	0.1	0.4	0.4	0.4	0.5	0.4
Other malignant neoplasms	6.5	5.5	3.3	4.8	4.7	2.2	3.6	2.3	3.7	6.1	3.3
Diabetes mellitus	2.1	0.7	0.8	0.4	0.9	0.2	1.6	1.0	0.8	1.5	0.7
Neuropsychiatric conditions	25.4	16.4	12.6	15.4	17.4	8.5	21.6	14.9	14.7	21.8	13.7
Unipolar major depression	6.8	5.0	5.6	7.3	6.6	3.5	6.4	6.0	5.7	6.1	5.6
Bipolar disorder	1.6	1.3	1.5	1.9	1.8	1.0	1.7	1.7	1.5	1.5	1.5
Schizophrenia	2.0	1.3	1.1	1.2	2.0	0.3	1.8	1.8	1.2	1.8	1.2
Alcohol use	4.5	2.7	0.6	0.8	1.8	1.3	5.6	0.3	1.7	3.8	1.4
Dementia and other CNS disorders	4.5	1.9	0.7	1.3	1.1	0.2	1.2	0.4	1.1	3.4	0.7
Drug use	1.4	0.8	0.0	0.1	0.8	0.3	1.5	1.1	0.6	1.2	0.5
Epilepsy	0.3	0.3	0.3	0.2	0.3	0.2	0.4	0.3	0.3	0.3	0.3
Other neuropsychiatric conditions	4.2	3.0	2.7	2.7	2.9	1.6	2.9	3.4	2.7	3.7	2.6
Glaucoma and cataracts	0.1	0.1	2.7	1.7	2.3	1.3	1.2	1.3	1.6	0.1	1.8
Cardiovascular diseases	19.4	26.1	18.4	16.3	15.6	6.0	13.2	17.7	14.7	22.0	13.8
Rheumatic heart disease	0.1	0.5	0.8	1.1	0.1	0.2	0.2	0.4	0.5	0.3	0.5
Ischemic heart disease	9.8	13.3	9.3	4.7	5.1	1.5	5.6	7.5	5.9	11.2	5.2
Cerebrovascular disease	5.1	7.7	3.4	8.2	4.5	2.6	4.3	2.8	4.4	6.2	4.2
Inflammatory heart diseases	0.6	0.7	1.0	0.6	1.2	0.6	0.6	1.4	0.8	0.6	0.9
Other cardiovascular diseases	3.7	3.8	4.0	1.6	4.7	1.1	2.5	5.6	3.1	3.7	3.0
Respiratory disease	5.3	8.1	6.4	16.3	4.3	4.5	6.3	6.6	7.3	6.4	7.4
Chronic obstructive pulmonary disease	2.9	3.3	2.8	14.5	1.7	1.4	2.5	2.2	4.1	3.1	4.3
Asthma	1.1	0.9	0.9	1.2	1.1	0.7	1.3	0.9	1.0	1.0	0.9
Other respiratory diseases	1.3	3.9	2.7	0.6	1.5	2.4	2.5	3.4	2.2	2.4	2.2
Digestive diseases	5.2	3.9	2.5	3.5	6.5	1.8	4.6	3.7	3.5	4.7	3.4
Cirrhosis of the liver	1.9	1.2	1.3	1.4	2.2	0.3	1.7	0.7	1.2	1.6	1.1
Other digestive diseases	3.2	2.7	1.2	2.1	4.3	1.5	2.9	3.0	2.3	3.0	2.3
Musculo-skeletal diseases	5.0	4.5	1.1	2.6	2.6	0.8	5.5	1.2	2.2	4.8	1.9
Rheumatoid arthritis	1.2	0.8	0.1	0.5	0.3	0.1	1.0	0.2	0.4	1.0	0.3
Osteoarthritis	3.5	3.4	1.0	1.9	2.2	0.7	4.2	0.9	1.7	3.5	1.5
Other musculo-skeletal diseases	0.4	0.2	0.0	0.2	0.2	0.0	0.3	0.1	0.1	0.3	0.1
Congential abnormalities	0.9	1.2	3.2	1.9	1.8	2.2	1.7	3.3	2.2	1.0	2.4
Oral conditions	1.0	0.8	0.8	0.7	1.5	0.3	1.3	1.8	0.9	0.9	0.9
Other noncommunicable diseases	2.9	1.7	0.9	1.6	1.8	1.9	2.8	2.9	1.9	2.4	1.8

Percentage of total DALYs[a]

Table 17. Burden of Disease, 2020 (*continued*)

Cause	Percentage of total DALYs[a]										
	EME	FSE	India	China	OAI	SSA	LAC	MEC	World	MDC	LDC
Injuries	10.1	17.4	19.1	16.4	17.2	28.3	19.3	20.5	20.1	13.0	21.1
Unintentional	6.9	11.6	16.4	11.0	13.6	15.4	13.2	9.8	13.0	8.8	13.6
Road-trafffic accidents	3.6	5.2	6.5	4.8	5.2	5.1	6.4	3.6	5.1	4.3	5.2
Poisoning	0.2	1.2	0.4	0.5	0.6	0.6	0.1	0.3	0.5	0.6	0.5
Falls	1.1	1.4	2.6	1.4	2.0	0.9	1.4	1.2	1.5	1.2	1.6
Fires	0.2	0.2	1.9	0.2	0.2	1.5	0.2	0.5	0.8	0.2	0.9
Drowning	0.2	0.7	0.8	1.0	1.1	1.2	0.7	0.7	0.9	0.4	1.0
Other unintentional injuries	1.6	2.9	4.2	3.1	4.5	5.9	4.3	3.4	4.2	2.1	4.4
Intentional injuries	3.2	5.7	2.8	5.4	3.6	12.9	6.2	10.7	7.1	4.2	7.5
Self-inflicted injuries	2.3	2.6	1.8	4.5	1.8	0.4	0.9	1.6	1.9	2.4	1.8
Violence	1.0	1.3	0.9	0.8	1.4	4.9	4.4	1.3	2.3	1.1	2.4
War	0.0	1.8	0.1	0.0	0.5	7.6	0.9	7.8	3.0	0.7	3.3
Other intentional injuries	0.0	0.0	0.0	0.0	0.0	0.0	0.0	0.0	0.0	0.0	0.0

EME: Established market economies.
FSE: Formerly socialist economies of Europe.
IOAI: Other Asia and islands (Asia, excluding Japan and Central Asia; Oceania, excluding Australia and New Zealand; and Indian Ocean islands).
SSA: Sub-Saharan Africa.
LAC: Latin America and the Caribbean.
MEC: Middle Eastern Crescent.
MDC: More-developed countries.
LDC: Less-developed countries.
a. DALYs are disability-adjusted life-years.

Table 18. Deaths by Age and Sex, 1990

				Male (Thousands)				Female			
	Total	Male	Female	0–4	5–14	15–59	60+	0–4	5–14	15–59	60+
Established Market Economies											
All causes	7,121	3,659	3,462	60	14	769	2,817	45	9	370	3,038
Communicable, maternal, perinatal, and nutritional conditions	453	237	216	31	1	51	155	22	1	15	179
Noncommunicable diseases	6,233	3,125	3,099	24	6	520	2,575	19	5	298	2,777
Injuries	445	298	147	6	7	197	88	4	3	57	81
Formerly Socialist Economies of Europe											
All causes	3,791	1,908	1,883	66	17	678	1,147	48	9	265	1,561
Communicable, maternal, perinatal, and nutritional conditions	214	109	105	38	1	24	45	27	1	8	69
Noncommunicable diseases	3,188	1,511	1,677	18	5	430	1,057	14	4	206	1,453
Injuries	389	288	101	9	11	223	44	7	5	50	39
India											
All causes	9,371	4,875	4,496	1,600	256	1,259	1,760	1,650	294	1,046	1,506
Communicable, maternal, perinatal, and nutritional conditions	4,775	2,418	2,356	1,411	129	445	435	1,479	171	411	295
Noncommunicable diseases	3,788	2,001	1,788	116	48	558	1,277	117	54	449	1,169
Injuries	808	456	352	73	79	256	48	55	69	187	41
China											
All causes	8,885	4,829	4,056	505	86	1,372	2,866	565	63	926	2,502
Communicable, maternal, perinatal, and nutritional conditions	11,405	708	697	342	16	125	225	399	17	110	171
Noncommunicable diseases	6,460	3,531	2,929	88	29	899	2,516	95	19	595	2,220
Injuries	1,020	590	430	75	42	348	125	71	27	222	111
Other Asia and Islands											
All causes	5,534	3,044	3,490	901	230	855	1,058	716	172	620	982
Communicable, maternal, perinatal, and nutritional conditions	2,190	1,161	1,029	747	82	150	182	586	72	205	166
Noncommunicable diseases	2,785	1,499	1,286	99	90	463	847	85	71	330	800
Injuries	559	384	175	54	58	242	29	45	28	85	17
Sub-Saharan Africa											
All causes	8,202	4,324	3,878	2,169	385	1,147	622	1,861	355	970	692
Communicable, maternal, perinatal, and nutritional conditions	5,316	2,671	2,645	2,008	203	313	149	1,720	213	550	161
Noncommunicable diseases	1,864	934	930	63	64	363	444	65	75	277	512
Injuries	1,022	718	303	98	118	471	30	76	67	142	17
Latin America and the Caribbean											
All causes	3,009	1,654	1,355	403	73	549	629	306	55	381	613
Communicable, maternal, perinatal, and nutritional conditions	943	511	432	340	19	86	66	251	22	95	63
Noncommunicable diseases	1,676	850	826	44	22	249	535	40	18	233	535
Injuries	398	293	97	19	32	214	29	14	15	53	15
Middle Eastern Crescent											
All causes	4,553	2,399	2,154	955	158	580	707	908	141	428	677
Communicable, maternal, perinatal, and nutritional conditions	1,945	980	964	789	46	67	77	752	46	100	65
Noncommunicable diseases	2,156	1,123	1,033	119	68	324	612	112	72	250	599
Injuries	452	296	156	46	44	189	17	44	23	78	12
World											
All causes	50,467	26,692	23,775	6,658	1,219	7,207	11,607	6,099	1,097	5,008	11,571
Communicable, maternal, perinatal, and nutritional conditions	17,241	8,796	8,445	5,705	496	1,262	1,333	5,236	543	1,495	1,170
Noncommunicable diseases	28,141	14,573	13,569	572	332	3,805	9,863	547	317	2,638	10,066
Injuries	5,084	3,323	1,761	381	390	2,141	411	238	196	428	234

Table 19. Deaths by Age and Sex, 2020

				Thousands							
				Male				Female			
	Total	Male	Female	0–4	5–14	15–59	60+	0–4	5–14	15–59	60+
Established Market Economies											
All causes	8,651	4,632	4,018	25	9	830	3,769	19	6	299	3,695
Communicable, maternal, perinatal, and nutritional conditions	533	299	234	12	0	74	213	8	0	13	213
Noncommunicable diseases	7,666	4,042	3,624	10	4	595	3,433	8	3	226	3,387
Injuries	451	291	160	3	4	160	124	3	3	61	95
Formerly Socialist Economies of Europe											
All causes	4,854	2,713	2,141	29	10	847	1,827	22	6	218	1,896
Communicable, maternal, perinatal, and nutritional conditions	140	65	75	12	0	7	46	9	0	2	65
Noncommunicable diseases	4,295	2,353	1,942	10	3	624	1,716	8	2	157	1,775
Injuries	419	295	123	6	7	218	65	5	4	59	56
India											
All causes	11,430	6,515	4,915	506	102	2,489	3,418	469	92	1,312	3,043
Communicable, maternal, perinatal, and nutritional conditions	2,461	1,402	1,059	348	25	577	452	332	28	356	343
Noncommunicable diseases	7,627	4,322	3,305	102	20	1,375	2,826	97	17	645	2,546
Injuries	1,085	644	441	51	53	417	122	34	42	224	141
China											
All causes	13,938	8,204	5,734	150	41	2,554	5,378	152	30	1,123	4,429
Communicable, maternal, perinatal, and nutritional conditions	540	285	255	62	1	21	201	64	2	14	175
Noncommunicable diseases	11,890	7,111	4,779	48	15	2,154	4,894	50	8	774	3,947
Injuries	1,508	809	699	40	24	460	283	38	20	335	306
Other Asia and Islands											
All causes	7,736	4,418	3,318	341	93	1,538	2,445	254	60	732	2,272
Communicable, maternal, perinatal, and nutritional conditions	1,105	587	518	229	15	122	220	165	12	106	234
Noncommunicable diseases	5,810	3,275	2,535	72	43	1,019	2,141	56	28	472	1,980
Injuries	822	556	265	39	36	397	84	33	20	154	57
Sub-Saharan Africa											
All causes	10,353	5,837	5,416	1,641	335	2,385	1,475	1,274	252	1,422	1,568
Communicable, maternal, perinatal, and nutritional conditions	4,014	2,111	1,903	1,350	92	467	202	1,034	96	557	216
Noncommunicable diseases	4,032	2,087	1,944	111	59	735	1,182	103	56	489	1,296
Injuries	2,307	1,638	669	180	185	1,181	92	137	99	376	56
Latin America and the Caribbean											
All causes	4,735	2,642	2,093	155	41	941	1,506	114	26	518	1,436
Communicable, maternal, perinatal, and nutritional conditions	519	308	211	112	4	99	92	78	4	36	91
Noncommunicable diseases	3,581	1,870	1,711	29	13	494	1,335	25	9	378	1,299
Injuries	636	464	171	14	24	348	79	11	13	102	45
Middle Eastern Crescent											
All causes	6,639	3,826	2,813	617	122	1,253	1,833	525	91	600	1,600
Communicable, maternal, perinatal, and nutritional conditions	992	530	462	408	13	30	78	352	12	25	73
Noncommunicable diseases	4,750	2,709	2,042	144	49	809	1,706	112	44	397	1,489
Injuries	896	587	309	64	60	414	49	61	34	177	38
World											
All causes	68,337	38,788	29,549	3,463	754	12,917	21,654	2,828	563	6,221	19,937
Communicable, maternal, perinatal, and nutritional conditions	10,305	5,588	4,717	2,535	151	1,397	1,505	2,043	156	1,108	1,411
Noncommunicable diseases	49,652	27,769	21,883	526	205	7,806	19,232	458	168	3,538	17,719
Injuries	8,381	5,432	2,949	403	397	3,715	917	328	239	1,576	807

Sources and Definitions

Aggregate Measures

For operational and analytical purposes, the World Bank's main criterion for classifying economies is gross national product (GNP) per capita. Every economy is classified as low income, middle income (subdivided into lower middle and upper middle), or high income. Historical data presented are based on the same country grouping using the most recent year for which GNP per capita data are available (1996). Low-income countries are those with GNP per capita of $785 or less in 1996. Middle-income economies are those with GNP per capita of more than $785 but less than $9,636. Lower-middle and upper-middle economies are separated at GNP per capita of $3,115. High-income economies are those with a GNP per capita of $9,636 or more.

The aggregate measures for regions include only low- and middle-income economies. The country composition of regions is based on the World Bank's operational regions and may differ from common geographic usage. See World Bank (1998), for regional classifications.

Also used are the terms "developing" or "less developed" and "developed" or "more developed" countries. In this classification, used by the United Nations, the former group includes all regions of Africa, Asia (excluding Japan), Latin America and the Caribbean, and Oceania (excluding Australia and New Zealand), and the latter includes North America, Japan, Europe (including the European successor states of the former USSR), Australia, and New Zealand. A .. indicates that data are not available.

Table 1. Health Expenditures, Basic Indicators

Total health expenditure, 1994 US$. This shows the total and per capita health expenditure in US$ millions at official exchange rates in 1994. Per capita health expenditure is also shown in PPP$ (purchasing power parity, or international prices). Data are given for the latest year in which they are relatively complete for both public and private expenditures.

Health expenditure as percentage of GDP (1990–95). This shows total, public, and private health expenditure as a percentage of GDP. The years for which the data are taken is indicated in the "year" column. *Public* health expenditure consists of spending from the following sources: government (local and central) budgets, external borrowings and grants, and social (or compulsory) health insurance funds. All external assistance, including donations from international NGOs, were included under the "public" expenditure category. *Private* health expenditure includes spending on health from the following sources: direct household expenditure (out-of-pocket), private insurance, charitable donations, and direct service payments by private corporations. Public expenditure is also shown as a percentage of total health expenditure.

Table 2. Health Expenditures, 1990–96

This table presents all of the available data on health expenditures as a percentage of GDP for 1990–96. Data for each country are not necessarily from the same source. Differences in the definition of health expenditure and in data collection methods between different sources are likely to introduce inconsistencies in some of the time series. Therefore, the time-series data should be interpreted with caution.

Table 3. Health Financing by Expenditure Categories

This table breaks down health financing by the following categories of expenditure: hospital, pharmaceuticals, capital investment, and personnel. Hospital and pharmaceutical expenditures are further disaggregated into total spending (public and private) and public spending. These categories comprise only a limited list of the major categories of expenditure, selected mainly on the basis of availability of data and the relatively consistent definition of these categories. Other important categories, such as research and development, medical education, and public health programs, will be added to future databases.

Table 4. Sources of Health Financing

This table disaggregates public health expenditures into sources of revenues. Public sources are divided into three main components: social health insurance (any form of publicly mandated and/or publicly managed insurance funds); government budget (from tax and other domestic sources of government revenues); and external assistance, in the form of either loans or grants. Public revenues from user charges, where available, are treated as "private" out-of-pocket payments.

Table 5. Health Services Indicators, 1990–95

Physicians per 1,000 population. Physicians include the total number of registered practitioners in the country. The definition of this differs among countries.

Inpatient beds per 1,000 population. Inpatient beds are defined as beds in public and private facilities where individuals receive medical care as inpatients. In most cases, beds for acute and chronic care are

included. The sources of the data in table 5 include government statistical yearbooks, World Health Organization (WHO), Pan American Health Organization (PAHO), Organisation for Economic Cooperation and Development (OECD), and World Bank country and sector reports.

Table 6. Utilization of Health Services, 1990–95

Outpatient visits. The number of annual visits to health care facilities per capita, including repeat visits.

Inpatient admissions. Percentage of population admitted to hospitals during a year.

Average length of stay. Average number of inpatient days per admission.

Bed occupancy rate. Average percentage of inpatient beds occupied during a year.

The sources of the data in table 6 are government statistical yearbooks, WHO, PAHO, OECD, and World Bank country and sector reports.

Table 7. Key Development Indicators

GNP per capita. This is calculated using the World Bank *Atlas* methodology, using midyear population estimates and the gross national product converted to U.S. dollars. Source: World Bank (1997c).

Gini coefficient. This index measures the extent to which the distribution of income among individuals or households deviates from a perfectly equal distribution. A Gini index of zero represents perfect equality while an index of 100 percent implies perfect inequality. Source: World Bank (1997c), based on household surveys conducted during 1990–95.

Population. Midyear estimates and projections of total de facto population. Refugees not permanently settled in the country of asylum are excluded from the estimates. Sources of population estimates vary from country to country and are based on the most recent census, official country estimates, UN Population Division estimates, or those of other international agencies. Projections are based on the cohort component methodology, in which a baseline age-sex structure is projected with fertility, mortality, and migration schedules. For a detailed description of the methodology and assumptions, see Bos and others (1995).

Population growth rates. These are average annual rates expressed in percentages, calculated from mid-year estimates and projections using an exponential rate of change.

Gross secondary school enrollment. The ratio of total enrollment, regardless of age, to the population of the age group that officially corresponds to the secondary level, which varies across countries. Source: World Bank (1997c).

Urban population. The percentage of a country's total population residing in urban areas. Definitions of urban areas are country-specific and vary considerably among countries. Source: United Nations (1994).

Crude birth rate and crude death rate. The number of births and deaths per 1,000 people. Estimates are based on national vital registration systems, demographic surveys, World Bank estimates, and those of other international organizations. A frequently used source is the UN Statistical Office's *Population and Vital Statistics Report* (issued quarterly).

Table 8. Child Mortality, 1960–95

Infant mortality rate. The number of deaths of infants under age one per 1,000 births. These are based on country statistical offices, censuses and surveys, World Bank sector studies and, especially for countries without reliable data, the UN Population Division's estimates. For many developing countries without reliable vital registration, indirect estimates from demographic surveys are used.

Children under five mortality rate. The probability that a newborn will survive to exactly age five, based on prevailing mortality rates, multiplied by 1,000. The estimates from 1960 to 1990 are based on a methodology developed by Hill and Yazbeck (1994) using regression analysis. Weighted least-square regression was used in their analysis, assigning weights to each country's data on the basis of the validity of the data. Figures for 1995 are World Bank staff estimates based on published sources such as UNICEF's (1997), and on

projections from the latest available survey, census, and vital registration data.

Table 9. Life Expectancy at Birth, 1960–95

Life expectancy at birth. The average number of years a newborn will live based on prevailing mortality rates. Note that by definition these are based on period life tables and may not apply to any cohort for which mortality conditions may be different in subsequent years. The sources for the data include the UN Population Division, national statistical offices, and World Bank estimates and projections from surveys and censuses. For most countries 1995 life expectancy estimates are projections based on the trend in the previous decade. HIV/AIDS prevalence data are used to adjust the trend and account for the declining life expectancy in countries where AIDS mortality is high.

Table 10. Adult Mortality, 1960–95

Adult mortality rate. The probability of dying between ages 15 and 60 based on prevailing mortality rates. For about 50 countries these are vital registration-based life table estimates; for other countries these are World Bank estimates based on model life tables selected on the basis of overall life expectancy (table 9) and morality rates for infants and children under five. For countries with vital registration-based life tables, a close fit between these model-based estimates and the life table values was found. However, such agreement cannot be assumed for all countries, and the data presented here should be interpreted as indicative of the level of adult mortality rather than as precise estimates.

Table 11. Total Fertility Rate, 1960–95

Total fertility rate. The average number of children born per woman entering childbearing age, if subject to prevailing fertility rates. The sources are the Demographic and Health Surveys, the World Fertility Surveys, the CDC Contraceptive Prevalence Surveys, other demographic surveys, vital registration, World Bank staff estimates, and the UN Population Division. As with some of the mortality data, estimates of past fertility are frequently based on indirect estimates from survey data.

Table 12. The Aging Population, 1995 and 2020

Percentage of population over age 60. The population of males and females that is age 60 or over, expressed as a percentage of the total number of males and total number of females. For 1995 these estimates are based on age structures from censuses, national statistical offices, or the UN Population Division. For 2020 these are projections based on trends in fertility, mortality, and migration, as described in Bos and others (1994).

Probability of surviving to age 60. These are period life table survival rates based on prevailing mortality rates, showing the percent of a cohort born in 1995 that would survive to at least age 60 if subject to prevailing mortality rates. As such, these are hypothetical, as mortality rates in the future are likely to be different from today's rate. If recent trends in mortality continue, a higher proportion of the 1995 birth cohort would reach age 60.

Table 13. Access to Safe Water, Sanitation, and Health Care

Access to safe water. The percentage of the population with access to safe water is the share of the population with reasonable access to an adequate amount of safe water, including treated surface water and untreated but uncontaminated well and spring water.

Access to sanitation. The percentage of the population with at least adequate excreta disposal facilities that can effectively prevent human, animal, and insect contact with excreta.

Access to health services. The percentage of the population covered for treatment of common diseases and injuries, including availability of essential drugs, within one hour's walk or travel. This indicator is limited to potential access to treatment and does not take other barriers (such as financial barriers) into account.

Immunization of children under 12 months for measles and DPT (diphtheria, pertussis, and tetanus). The percentage of children under 12 months of age that are immunized against measles (one dose of vaccine) and DPT (at least two of three doses of vaccine). The source for data in table 13 is World Bank (1997c), based on and supplemented by data collected by WHO and UNICEF.

Table 14. Other Health Determinants and Outcomes

Child malnutrition rate. The prevalence of malnutrition is measured as the percentage of children under five whose weight for their age is less than minus two standard deviations from the median of the reference population. The data are mostly from WHO, *World Health Statistics Annual,* supplemented with data from UNICEF and the United Nations.

Anemia among pregnant women. The percentage of pregnant women whose hemoglobin is less than 11 grams per deciliter. Data are mostly from surveys during 1980–95, as reported by WHO.

Prevalence of low birth weight babies. The percentage of children born weighing less than 2,500 grams, with the measurement taken within the first hours of life, before significant postnatal weight loss has occurred. Data are mostly from WHO, supplemented with data from UNICEF.

Prevalence of obesity. The percentage of the population with a body mass index of 30 or higher. Data denoted (a) are for children; data denoted (b) are for adults. Sources for the data are the FAO and the Demographic and Health Surveys.

Dietary energy supply (kcal/day). The number of kilocalories (kcal) consumed a day per person. The data are from the FAO (1996).

Tuberculosis incidence. The estimated number of new sputum smear positive (SS+) cases per 100,000 population. Source: WHO (1997).

Percentage of kcal from fat. The percentage of total kilocalories from fat.

Smoking prevalence. Percentage of males and females over age 15 who smoke tobacco products. Sources are WHO and World Bank country surveys for the most recently available year.

Table 15. Reproductive Health Indicators

Maternal mortality ratio. The number of deaths of women during pregnancy and childbirth per 100,000 live births in the same year. The estimates are from the Demographic and Health Surveys, national estimates, and, for countries without such data, from a model developed by WHO and UNICEF that is based on fertility and other variables related to maternal mortality. The measurement of maternal mortality is often inaccurate due to underreporting in vital registration, large standard errors in survey-based estimates, and the use of indirect methods that produce estimates for past years. All maternal mortality estimates, but especially the model-based figures, should be seen as indicative of the magnitude of the problem.

Adolescent fertility rate. The fertility rate for women under age 20, shown per 1,000 women under age 20. These are estimates and projections based on Demographic and Health Surveys, national estimates, and other sources of age-specific fertility rates. For some countries that lack age-specific fertility schedules, the figures are based on models.

Contraceptive prevalence rate. The percentage of married women (or their husbands) using any type of contraceptive method. The source is mainly the Demographic and Health Survey program, supplemented with other survey data and national estimates. Family planning program statistics are not used, as these tend to overestimate contraceptive use.

Adult HIV prevalence. The percentage of those over age 15 who are HIV positive. Source: UNAIDS, based on blood screening of pregnant women, blood donors, and the general population.

Percentage of births attended by health staff. The percentage of deliveries attended by personnel trained to give the necessary supervision, care, and advice to women during labor and the postpartum period, to conduct deliveries on their own, and to care for the newborn and the infant. Source: World Bank (1997c), based on data from WHO.

Tables 16 and 17. Burden of Disease, 1990 and 2020

These tables for 1990 and 2020 show the burden of disease by disease and injury categories for the world, for more developed countries, for less developed countries, and for eight regions (as defined in World Bank (1993)). The burden of disease is measured in number of DALYs (disability-adjusted life-years) lost to the specified cause, which allows for a quantitative comparison of the disease burden in different regions and for different causes. The estimates and projections shown are from Murray and Lopez (1996a), which also provides the methodological details. It should be recognized that the estimates for 1990 are based on very limited empirical data and required broad generalizations on the part of the authors. The projections for 2020 are by definition hypothetical and should be interpreted as the calculated outcomes of the assumptions about changing disease patterns applied to assumptions about changing age structures.

Tables 18 and 19. Deaths by Age and Sex, 1990 and 2020

These tables show the number of deaths by broad cause, by age group and sex, for the same regions as in the previous two tables. The data are from Murray and Lopez (1996a). Methodological details and caveats about the figures can also be found in this volume.

References

Abel-Smith, Brian. 1963. *Paying for Health Services.* Public Health Papers 17. Geneva: World Health Organization.

———. 1967. *An International Study of Health Expenditure.* Public Health Papers No. 32. Geneva: World Health Organization.

Bos, Eduard, M. T. Vu, E. Massiah, R. Bulatao. 1994. *World Population Projections, 1994-95.* Baltimore: The Johns Hopkins University Press.

Chellaray, Gnanaraj, O. Adeyi, A. Preker, E. Goldstein. 1996. *Trends in Health Status, Services, and Finance: The Transition in Central and Eastern Europe.* World Bank Technical Paper 348. Washington, D.C.

FAO (Food and Agriculture Organization). 1996. *Sixth World Food Survey, 1996.* Rome.

Hill, Kenneth, and Abdo Yazbeck. 1994. "Trends in Child Mortality 1960–90." Background Paper Series No. 6, World Development Report 1993. World Bank, Washington, D.C.

Murray, Christopher, and A. Lopez, eds. 1996a. *The Global Burden of Disease.* Harvard School of Public Health for the World Health Organization and the World Bank. Cambridge, Mass.: Harvard University Press.

———. 1996b. *Global Health Statistics.* Harvard School of Public Health for the World Health Organization and the World Bank. Cambridge, Mass.: Harvard University Press.

UNICEF (United Nations Children's Fund). 1997. *State of the World's Children.* New York.

United Nations, Population Division. 1994. *World Urbanization Prospects.* New York.

Untied Nations, Statistical Office. Quarterly. *Population and Vital Statistics Report.* New York.

World Bank. 1993. *World Development Report 1993: Investing in Health.* New York: Oxford University Press.

———. 1997a. *Health, Nutrition, and Population Sector Strategy.* Washington, D.C.

———. 1997b. *World Development Indicators 1997.* Washington, D.C.

———. 1997c. *World Development Report 1997: The State in a Changing World.* New York: Oxford University Press.

———. 1998. *World Development Indicators 1998.* Washington, D.C.

WHO (World Health Organization). Various years. *World Health Statistics Annual.* Geneva.

———. 1997. *Global Tuberculosis Control Report.* Geneva.

Distributors of World Bank Publications

Prices and credit terms vary from country to country. Consult your local distributor before placing an order.

ARGENTINA
World Publications SA
Av. Cordoba 1877
1120 Ciudad de Buenos Aires
Tel: (54 11) 4815-8156
Fax: (54 11) 4815-8156
E-mail: wpbooks@infovia.com.ar

AUSTRALIA, FIJI, PAPUA NEW GUINEA, SOLOMON ISLANDS, VANUATU, AND SAMOA
D.A. Information Services
648 Whitehorse Road
Mitcham 3132
Victoria
Tel: (61) 3 9210 7777
Fax: (61) 3 9210 7788
E-mail: service@dadirect.com.au
URL: http://www.dadirect.com.au

AUSTRIA
Gerold and Co.
Weihburggasse 26
A-1011 Wien
Tel: (43 1) 512-47-31-0
Fax: (43 1) 512-47-31-29
URL: http://www.gerold.co/at.online

BANGLADESH
Micro Industries Development
    Assistance Society (MIDAS)
House 5, Road 16
Dhanmondi R/Area
Dhaka 1209
Tel: (880 2) 326427
Fax: (880 2) 811188

BELGIUM
Jean De Lannoy
Av. du Roi 202
1060 Brussels
Tel: (32 2) 538-5169
Fax: (32 2) 538-0841

BRAZIL
Publicacoes Tecnicas Internacionais Ltda.
Rua Peixoto Gomide, 209
01409 Sao Paulo, SP.
Tel: (55 11) 259-6644
Fax: (55 11) 258-6990
E-mail: postmaster@pti.uol.br
URL: http://www.uol.br

CANADA
Renouf Publishing Co. Ltd.
5369 Canotek Road
Ottawa, Ontario K1J 9J3
Tel: (613) 745-2665
Fax: (613) 745-7660
E-mail: order.dept@renoufbooks.com
URL: http://www.renoufbooks.com

CHINA
China Financial & Economic Publishing
House
8, Da Fo Si Dong Jie
Beijing
Tel: (86 10) 6401-7365
Fax: (86 10) 6401-7365

China Book Import Centre
P.O. Box 2825
Beijing

Chinese Corporation for Promotion of
Humanities
52 You Fang Hu Tong,
Xuan Nei Da Jie
Beijing
Tel: (86 10) 660 72 494
Fax: (86 10) 660 72 494

COLOMBIA
Infoenlace Ltda.
Carrera 6 No. 51-21
Apartado Aereo 34270
Santafé de Bogotá, D.C.
Tel: (57 1) 285-2798
Fax: (57 1) 285-2798

COTE D'IVOIRE
Center d'Edition et de Diffusion Africaines
(CEDA)
04 B.P. 541
Abidjan 04
Tel: (225) 24 6510; 24 6511
Fax: (225) 25 0567

CYPRUS
Center for Applied Research
Cyprus College
6, Diogenes Street, Engomi
P.O. Box 2006
Nicosia
Tel: (357 2) 59-0730
Fax: (357 2) 66-2051

CZECH REPUBLIC
USIS, NIS Prodejna
Havelkova 22
130 00 Prague 3
Tel: (420 2) 2423 1486
Fax: (420 2) 2423 1114
URL: http://www.nis.cz/

DENMARK
SamfundsLitteratur
Rosenoerns Allé 11
DK-1970 Frederiksberg C
Tel: (45 35) 351942
Fax: (45 35) 357822
URL: http://www.sl.cbs.dk

ECUADOR
Libri Mundi
Libreria Internacional
P.O. Box 17-01-3029
Juan Leon Mera 851
Quito
Tel: (593 2) 521-606; (593 2) 544-185
Fax: (593 2) 504-209
E-mail: librimu1@librimundi.com.ec
E-mail: librimu2@librimundi.com.ec

CODEU
Ruiz de Castilla 763, Edif. Expocolor
Primer piso, Of. #2
Quito
Tel/Fax: (593 2) 507-383; 253-091
E-mail: codeu@impsat.net.ec

EGYPT, ARAB REPUBLIC OF
Al Ahram Distribution Agency
Al Galaa Street
Cairo
Tel: (20 2) 578-6083
Fax: (20 2) 578-6833

The Middle East Observer
41, Sherif Street
Cairo
Tel: (20 2) 393-9732
Fax: (20 2) 393-9732

FINLAND
Akateeminen Kirjakauppa
P.O. Box 128
FIN-00101, Helsinki
Tel: (358 0) 121 4418
Fax: (358 0) 121-4435
E-mail: akatilaus@stockmann.fi
URL: http://www.akateeminen.com

FRANCE
Editions Eska; DBJ
48, rue Gay Lussac
75005 Paris
Tel: (33-1) 55-42-73-08
Fax: (33-1) 43-29-91-67

GERMANY
UNO-Verlag
Poppelsdorfer Allee 55
53115 Bonn

Tel: (49 228) 949020
Fax: (49 228) 217492
URL: http://www.uno-verlag.de
E-mail: unoverlag@aol.com

GHANA
Epp Books Services
P.O. Box 44
TUC
Accra
Tel: 223 21 778843
Fax: 223 21 779099

GREECE
Papasotiriou S.A.
35, Stournara Str.
106 82 Athens
Tel: (30 1) 364-1826
Fax: (30 1) 364-8254

HAITI
Culture Diffusion
5, Rue Capois
C.P. 257
Port-au-Prince
Tel: (509) 23 9260
Fax: (509) 23 4858

HONG KONG, CHINA; MACAO
Asia 2000 Ltd.
Sales & Circulation Department
302 Seabird House
22-28 Wyndham Street, Central
Hong Kong, China
Tel: (852) 2530-1409
Fax: (852) 2526-1107
E-mail: sales@asia2000.com.hk
URL: http://www.asia2000.com.hk

HUNGARY
Euro Info Service
Margitszgeti Europa Haz
H-1138 Budapest
Tel: (36 1) 350 80 24, 350 80 25
Fax: (36 1) 350 90 32
E-mail: euroinfo@mail.matav.hu

INDIA
Allied Publishers Ltd.
751 Mount Road
Madras - 600 002
Tel: (91 44) 852-3938
Fax: (91 44) 852-0649

INDONESIA
Pt. Indira Limited
Jalan Borobudur 20
P.O. Box 181
Jakarta 10320
Tel: (62 21) 390-4290
Fax: (62 21) 390-4289

IRAN
Ketab Sara Co. Publishers
Khaled Eslamboli Ave., 6th Street
Delafrooz Alley No. 8
P.O. Box 15745-733
Tehran 15117
Tel: (98 21) 8717819; 8716104
Fax: (98 21) 8712479
E-mail: ketab-sara@neda.net.ir

Kowkab Publishers
P.O. Box 19575-511
Tehran
Tel: (98 21) 258-3723
Fax: (98 21) 258-3723

IRELAND
Government Supplies Agency
Oifig an tSoláthair
4-5 Harcourt Road
Dublin 2
Tel: (353 1) 661-3111
Fax: (353 1) 475-2670

ISRAEL
Yozmot Literature Ltd.
P.O. Box 56055
3 Yohanan Hasandlar Street
Tel Aviv 61560

Tel: (972 3) 5285-397
Fax: (972 3) 5285-397

R.O.Y. International
PO Box 13056
Tel Aviv 61130
Tel: (972 3) 649 9469
Fax: (972 3) 648 6039
E-mail: royil@netvision.net.il

Palestinian Authority/Middle East
Index Information Services
P.O.B. 19502 Jerusalem
Tel: (972 2) 6271219
Fax: (972 2) 6271634

ITALY, LIBERIA
Licosa Commissionaria Sansoni SPA
Via Duca Di Calabria, 1/1
Casella Postale 552
50125 Firenze
Tel: (39 55) 645-415
Fax: (39 55) 641-257
E-mail: licosa@ftbcc.it
URL: http://www.ftbcc.it/licosa

JAMAICA
Ian Randle Publishers Ltd.
206 Old Hope Road, Kingston 6
Tel: 876-927-2085
Fax: 876-977-0243
E-mail: irpl@colis.com

JAPAN
Eastern Book Service
3-13 Hongo 3-chome, Bunkyo-ku
Tokyo 113
Tel: (81 3) 3818-0861
Fax: (81 3) 3818-0864
E-mail: orders@svt-ebs.co.jp
URL: http://www.bekkoame.or.jp/~svt-ebs

KENYA
Africa Book Service (E.A.) Ltd.
Quaran House, Mfangano Street
P.O. Box 45245
Nairobi
Tel: (254 2) 223 641
Fax: (254 2) 330 272

Legacy Books
Loita House
Mezzanine 1
P.O. Box 68077
Nairobi
Tel: (254) 2-330853, 221426
Fax: (254) 2-330854, 561654
E-mail: Legacy@form-net.com

KOREA, REPUBLIC OF
Dayang Books Trading Co.
International Division
783-20, Pangba Bon-Dong, Socho-ku
Seoul
Tel: (82 2) 536-9555
Fax: (82 2) 536-0025
E-mail: seamap@chollian.net

Eulyoo Publishing Co., Ltd.
46-1, Susong-Dong, Jongro-Gu
Seoul
Tel: (82 2) 734-3515
Fax: (82 2) 732-9154

LEBANON
Librairie du Liban
P.O. Box 11-9232
Beirut
Tel: (961 9) 217 944
Fax: (961 9) 217 434
E-mail: hsayegh@librairie-du-liban.com.lb
URL: http://www.librairie-du-liban.com.lb

MALAYSIA
University of Malaya Cooperative
    Bookshop, Limited
P.O. Box 1127
Jalan Pantai Baru
59700 Kuala Lumpur
Tel: (60 3) 756-5000
Fax: (60 3) 755-4424
E-mail: umkoop@tm.net.my

MEXICO
INFOTEC
Av. San Fernando No. 37
Col. Toriello Guerra
14050 Mexico, D.F.
Tel: (52 5) 624-2800
Fax: (52 5) 624-2822
E-mail: infotec@rtn.net.mx
URL: http://rtn.net.mx

Mundi-Prensa Mexico S.A. de C.V.
c/Rio Panuco, 141-Colonia Cuauhtemoc
06500 Mexico, D.F.
Tel: (52 5) 533-5658
Fax: (52 5) 514-6799

NEPAL
Everest Media International Services (P.) Ltd.
GPO Box 5443
Kathmandu
Tel: (977 1) 416 026
Fax: (977 1) 224 431

NETHERLANDS
De Lindeboom/Internationale Publicaties
b.v.-
P.O. Box 202, 7480 AE Haaksbergen
Tel: (31 53) 574-0004
Fax: (31 53) 572-9296
E-mail: lindeboo@worldonline.nl
URL: http://www.worldonline.nl/~lindeboo

NEW ZEALAND
EBSCO NZ Ltd.
Private Mail Bag 99914
New Market
Auckland
Tel: (64 9) 524-8119
Fax: (64 9) 524-8067

Oasis Official
P.O. Box 3627
Wellington
Tel: (64 4) 499 1551
Fax: (64 4) 499 1972
E-mail: oasis@actrix.gen.nz
URL: http://www.oasisbooks.co.nz/

NIGERIA
University Press Limited
Three Crowns Building Jericho
Private Mail Bag 5095
Ibadan
Tel: (234 22) 41-1356
Fax: (234 22) 41-2056

PAKISTAN
Mirza Book Agency
65, Shahrah-e-Quaid-e-Azam
Lahore 54000
Tel: (92 42) 735 3601
Fax: (92 42) 576 3714

Oxford University Press
5 Bangalore Town
Sharae Faisal
PO Box 13033
Karachi-75350
Tel: (92 21) 446307
Fax: (92 21) 4547640
E-mail: ouppak@TheOffice.net

Pak Book Corporation
Aziz Chambers 21, Queen's Road
Lahore
Tel: (92 42) 636 3222, 636 0885
Fax: (92 42) 636 2328

PERU
Editorial Desarrollo SA
Apartado 3824, Ica 242 OF. 106
Lima 1
Tel: (51 14) 285380
Fax: (51 14) 286628

PHILIPPINES
International Booksource Center Inc.
1127-A Antipolo St, Barangay, Venezuela
Makati City
Tel: (63 2) 896 6501; 6505; 6507
Fax: (63 2) 896 1741

POLAND
International Publishing Service
Ul. Piekna 31/37
00-677 Warzawa
Tel: (48 2) 628-6089
Fax: (48 2) 621-7255
E-mail: books%ips@ikp.atm.com.pl
URL: http://www.ipscg.waw.pl/ips/export/

PORTUGAL
Livraria Portugal
Apartado 2681, Rua Do Carmo 70-74
1200 Lisbon
Tel: (1) 347-4982
Fax: (1) 347-0264

ROMANIA
Compani De Librarii Bucuresti S.A.
Str. Lipscani no. 26, sector 3
Bucharest
Tel: (40 1) 313 9645
Fax: (40 1) 312 4000

RUSSIAN FEDERATION
Isdatelstvo <Ves Mir>
9a, Kolpachniy Pereulok
Moscow 101831
Tel: (7 095) 917 87 49
Fax: (7 095) 917 92 59

**SINGAPORE; TAIWAN, CHINA
MYANMAR; BRUNEI**
Hemisphere Publication Services
41 Kallang Pudding Road #04-03
Golden Wheel Building
Singapore 349316
Tel: (65) 741-5166
Fax: (65) 742-9356
E-mail: ashgate@asianconnect.com

SLOVENIA
Gospodarski vestnik Publishing Group
Dunajska cesta 5
1000 Ljubljana
Tel: (386 61) 133 83 47; 132 12 30
Fax: (386 61) 133 80 30
E-mail: repansekj@gvestnik.si

SOUTH AFRICA, BOTSWANA
For single titles:
Oxford University Press Southern Africa
Vasco Boulevard, Goodwood
P.O. Box 12119, N1 City 7463
Cape Town
Tel: (27 21) 595 4400
Fax: (27 21) 595 4430
E-mail: oxford@oup.co.za

For subscription orders:
International Subscription Service
P.O. Box 41095
Craighall
Johannesburg 2024
Tel: (27 11) 880-1448
Fax: (27 11) 880-6248
E-mail: iss@is.co.za

SPAIN
Mundi-Prensa Libros, S.A.
Castello 37
28001 Madrid
Tel: (34 91) 4 363700
Fax: (34 91) 5 753998
E-mail: libreria@mundiprensa.es
URL: http://www.mundiprensa.es/

Mundi-Prensa Barcelona
Consell de Cent, 391
08009 Barcelona
Tel: (34 3) 488-3492
Fax: (34 3) 487-7659
E-mail: barcelona@mundiprensa.es

SRI LANKA, THE MALDIVES
Lake House Bookshop
100, Sir Chittampalam Gardiner Mawatha
Colombo 2
Tel: (94 1) 32105
Fax: (94 1) 432104
E-mail: LHL@sri.lanka.net

SWEDEN
Wennergren-Williams AB
P.O. Box 1305
S-171 25 Solna
Tel: (46 8) 705-97-50
Fax: (46 8) 27-00-71
E-mail: mail@wwi.se

SWITZERLAND
Librairie Payot Service Institutionnel
Cîtes-de-Montbenon 30
1002 Lausanne
Tel: (41 21) 341-3229
Fax: (41 21) 341-3235

ADECO Van Diermen EditionsTechniques
Ch. de Lacuez 41
CH1807 Blonay
Tel: (41 21) 943 2673
Fax: (41 21) 943 3605

THAILAND
Central Books Distribution
306 Silom Road
Bangkok 10500
Tel: (66 2) 2336930-9
Fax: (66 2) 237-8321

**TRINIDAD & TOBAGO
AND THE CARRIBBEAN**
Systematics Studies Ltd.
St. Augustine Shopping Center
Eastern Main Road, St. Augustine
Trinidad & Tobago, West Indies
Tel: (868) 645-8466
Fax: (868) 645-8467
E-mail: tobe@trinidad.net

UGANDA
Gustro Ltd.
PO Box 9997, Madhvani Building
Plot 16/4 Jinja Rd.
Kampala
Tel: (256 41) 251 467
Fax: (256 41) 251 468
E-mail: gus@swiftuganda.com

UNITED KINGDOM
Microinfo Ltd.
P.O. Box 3, Omega Park, Alton,
Hampshire GU34 2PG
England
Tel: (44 1420) 86848
Fax: (44 1420) 89889
E-mail: wbank@microinfo.co.uk
URL: http://www.microinfo.co.uk

The Stationery Office
51 Nine Elms Lane
London SW8 5DR
Tel: (44 171) 873-8400
Fax: (44 171) 873-8242
URL: http://www.theso.co.uk/

VENEZUELA
Tecni-Ciencia Libros, S.A.
Centro Cuidad Comercial Tamanco
Nivel C2, Caracas
Tel: (58 2) 959 5547, 5035, 0016
Fax: (58 2) 959 5636

ZAMBIA
University Bookshop, University of Zambia
Great East Road Campus
P.O. Box 32379
Lusaka
Tel: (260 1) 252 576
Fax: (260 1) 255 952

ZIMBABWE
Academic and Baobab Books (Pvt.) Ltd.
4 Conald Road, Graniteside
P.O. Box 567
Harare
Tel: 263 4 755035
Fax: 263 4 781913